Basic Statistics
and Epidemiology
A Practical Guide

FOURTH EDITION

Basic Statistics
and Epidemiology
A Practical Guide

FOURTH EDITION

Antony Stewart FFPH

Professor in Public Health at Staffordshire University;
Honorary Consultant in Public Health at Public Health England;
Clinical Research Specialty Lead for Public Health at NIHR
Clinical Research Network: West Midlands; and Academic
Director of the Centre for Health and Development (CHAD), UK

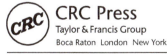
CRC Press
Taylor & Francis Group
Boca Raton London New York

CRC Press is an imprint of the
Taylor & Francis Group, an **informa** business

CRC Press
Taylor & Francis Group
6000 Broken Sound Parkway NW, Suite 300
Boca Raton, FL 33487-2742

© 2016 by Antony Stewart
CRC Press is an imprint of Taylor & Francis Group, an Informa business

No claim to original U.S. Government works

Printed on acid-free paper
Version Date: 20160106

International Standard Book Number-13: 978-1-78523-116-2 (Paperback)

Visit the Taylor & Francis Web site at
http://www.taylorandfrancis.com

and the CRC Press Web site at
http://www.crcpress.com

Contents

Preface to fourth edition

This book is offered as a basic primer in basic statistics and epidemiology, and focuses on their practical use rather than just theory.

The topics are relevant to a wide range of health professionals, students and anyone with an interest in medical statistics, public health, epidemiology, healthcare evaluation or who just needs to refresh previous learning.

It is aimed at people who want to grasp the main issues with minimum fuss. With this in mind, the avoidance of too much detail has been crucial. After reading this book, however, you might want to find further publications that give more detail, to enhance your knowledge. With this in mind, a further reading section has been added near the end.

This edition has been updated and includes new chapters on data checking and effect size, and an updated evidence-based healthcare section. Two new exercises have also been added, allowing you to further test your understanding. The chapters and exercises use practical examples, and full step-by-step instructions have been provided for most calculations.

I realised a long time ago that no single book can match everyone's individual learning style, so I cannot realistically **promise** that you will like it. But I have tried to produce a book that is accessible, using plain language and assuming no previous statistical knowledge. For this reason, I hope it will have some significance for you!

Antony Stewart
December 2015

Acknowledgements

I am grateful to the following organisations and individuals who have granted permission to reproduce their material in this book: Dr Florian Fritzsche and *BMC Public Health* (Figures 4.1 and 4.2), the *BMJ* (Figure 4.3; Tables 26.3 and 26.4), the Royal Society for Public Health (Figure 12.1; Table 20.1), Professor Sir Liam Donaldson and Radcliffe Publishing (Figures 29.1 and 30.1), the UK National Screening Committee (the screening criteria in Chapter 32), Professor Douglas Altman (the statistical tables in Appendix 1), Professor Douglas Altman and Wiley-Blackwell (the nomogram in Chapter 21), the Critical Appraisal Skills Programme (CASP) (*10 Questions to Help You Make Sense of a Review*, which appears in Chapter 33), Dr Andrew Moore of *Bandolier* (the material on logistic regression in Chapter 19) and Professor Rollin Brant (the online sample size calculator (Chapter 21)).

In addition to those who provided comments on previous editions, my sincere thanks also go to friends and colleagues who kindly read and commented on sections of this fourth edition prior to publication, including Dr Belinda Barton, Professor Tom Cochrane, Julie Hadley, Simon Hailstone, Dr Rachel Jordan, Dr Jennifer Peat and Dr Aviva Petrie.

Special thanks go to David Goda, who has provided generous friendship and advice on all four editions – and promptly answered all my queries, even when they were sent late on a Sunday evening!

This book is dedicated to Jenny, Katie and Michael,
and to the memory of my father, Jozef Stewart (1918–1984)
and mother, Edith Stewart (1923–2011).

CHAPTER 1

What are statistics?

1. Antibiotics reduce the duration of viral throat infections by 1–2 days.
2. Five per cent of women aged 30–49 consult their GP each year with heavy menstrual bleeding.
3. At our health centre, 50 patients were diagnosed with angina last year.

(after Rowntree, 1981)

The above quotes may be fact or fallacy, but they are familiar examples of **statistics**. We use statistics every day, often without realising it. Statistics as an academic study has been defined as follows:

> The science of assembling and interpreting numerical data (Bland, 2000)

> The discipline concerned with the treatment of numerical data derived from groups of individuals (Armitage *et al.*, 2001)

The term **data** refers to 'items of information', and is plural. When we use statistics to describe data, they are called **descriptive statistics**. All of the above three statements are descriptive.

However, as well as just describing data, statistics can be used to **draw conclusions** or to **make predictions** about what may happen in other subjects. This can apply to small groups of people or objects, or to whole populations. A **population** is a complete set of people or other subjects which can be studied. A **sample** is a smaller part of that population. For example, 'all the smokers in the UK' can be regarded as a population. In a study on smoking, it would be almost impossible to study every single smoker. We might therefore choose to study a smaller group of, say, 1000 smokers. These 1000 smokers would be our sample.

When we are using statistics to draw conclusions about a whole population using results from our samples, or to make predictions of what will happen, they are called

inferential statistics. Statements 1 and 2 on page 1 are examples of inferential statistics. It is important to recognise that when we use statistics in this way, we never know exactly what the true results in the population will be. For example, we shall never know how often every woman consults her GP (these data are not routinely collected in primary care at present), but we can draw a conclusion that is based on a sample of data.

A **statistic** is a quantity calculated from a **sample**, which describes a particular feature. Statistics are always estimates. The true quantities of the **population** (which are rarely known for certain) are called **parameters**.

Different types of data and information call for different types of statistics. Some of the commonest situations are described on the following pages.

Before we go any further, a word about the use of computers and formulae in statistics. There are several excellent computer software packages (as well as calculators) that can perform statistical calculations more or less automatically. Some of these packages are available free of charge, while some cost well over £1000. Each package has its own merits, and careful consideration is required before deciding which one to use. These packages can avoid the need to work laboriously through formulae, and are especially useful when one is dealing with large samples. However, care must be taken when interpreting computer outputs, as will be demonstrated later by the example in Chapter 6. Also, computers can sometimes allow one to perform statistical tests that are inappropriate. For this reason, it is vital to understand factors such as the following:

- which statistical test should be performed
- why it is being performed
- what type of data are appropriate
- how to interpret the results.

Several formulae appear on the following pages, some of which look fairly horrendous. Don't worry too much about these – you may never actually need to work them out by hand. However, you may wish to work through a few examples in order to get a 'feel' for how they work in practice. Working through the exercises in Appendix 2 will also help you. Remember, though, that the application of statistics and the interpretation of the results obtained are what really matter.

CHAPTER 2

Populations and samples

It is important to understand the difference between populations and samples. You will remember from the previous chapter that a **population** can be defined as **every subject** in a country, a town, a district or other group being studied. Imagine that you are conducting a study of post-operative infection rates in a hospital during 2014. The population for your study (called the **target population**) is **everyone** in that hospital who underwent surgery during 2014. Using this population, a **sampling frame** can be constructed. This is a list of every person in the population from whom your sample will be taken. Each individual in the sampling frame is usually assigned a number, which can be used in the actual sampling process.

If thousands of operations have been performed during 2014, there may not be time to look at every case history. It may therefore only be possible to look at a smaller group (e.g. 200) of these patients. This smaller group is a **sample**.

Remember that a **statistic** is a value calculated from a **sample**, which describes a particular feature. This means it is always an **estimate** of the true value.

If we take a sample of 100 patients who underwent surgery during 2014, we might find that 7 patients developed a post-operative infection. However, a different sample of 100 patients might identify 11 post-operative infections, and yet another might find 8 infections. We shall almost always find such differences between samples, and these are called **sampling variations**.

When undertaking a scientific study, the aim is usually to be able to generalise the results to the population as a whole. Therefore we need a sample that is **representative** of the population. Going back to our example of post-operative infections, it is rarely possible to collect data on everyone in a population. Methods therefore exist for collecting sufficient data to be reasonably certain that the results will be accurate and applicable to the whole population. The random sampling methods that are described in the next chapter are among those used to achieve this.

Thus we usually have to rely on a sample for a study, because it may not be practicable to collect data from **everyone** in the population. A sample can be used to

estimate quantities in the population as a whole, and to calculate the likely accuracy of the estimate.

Many sampling techniques exist, and these can be divided into **non-random** and **random** techniques. In random sampling (also called **probability sampling**), everyone in the sampling frame has an equal probability of being chosen. This approach aims to make the sample more representative of the population from which it is drawn. There are several methods of random sampling, some of which are discussed in the next chapter. Non-random sampling (also called **non-probability sampling**) does not have these aims, but is usually easier and more convenient to perform.

Convenience or **opportunistic sampling** is the crudest type of non-random sampling. This involves selecting the most convenient group available (e.g. using the first 20 colleagues you see at work). It is simple to perform, but is unlikely to result in a sample that is either representative of the population or replicable.

A commonly used **non-random** method of sampling is **quota sampling**, in which a predefined number (or quota) of people who meet certain criteria are surveyed. For example, an interviewer may be given the task of interviewing 25 women with toddlers in a town centre on a weekday morning, and the instructions may specify that seven of these women should be aged under 30 years, ten should be aged between 30 and 45 years, and eight should be aged over 45 years. While this is a convenient sampling method, it may not produce results that are representative of all women with children of toddler age. For instance, the described example will systematically exclude women who are in full-time employment.

As well as using the correct method of sampling, there are also ways of calculating a sample size that is appropriate. This is important, since increasing the sample size will tend to increase the accuracy of your estimate, while a smaller sample size will usually decrease the accuracy. Furthermore, the right sample size is essential to enable you to detect a real effect, if one exists. The appropriate sample size can be calculated using one of several formulae, according to the type of study and the type of data being collected. The basic elements of sample size calculation are discussed in Chapter 21. Sample size calculation should generally be left to a statistician or someone with a good knowledge of the requirements and procedures involved. If statistical significance is not essential, a sample size of between 50 and 100 may suffice for many purposes.

CHAPTER 3

Random sampling

Random selection of samples is another important issue. In random sampling, everyone in the sampling frame has an equal probability of being chosen. For a sample to be truly representative of the population, a random sample should be taken. Random sampling can also help to minimise **bias**. Bias can be defined as an effect that produces results which are **systematically** different from the **true** values (*see* Chapter 24).

For example, imagine that you are conducting a study on hypertension (high blood pressure). You have 300 hypertensive patients, and want to find out what proportion have had their blood pressure checked in the past year. You might make a list of all of these patients, and decide to examine the records of the first 50 patients on the list. If most of them are found to have received blood pressure checks, are the other 250 patients likely to be similar? Furthermore, what if someone accuses you of 'fixing' the sample by only selecting patients who you know have received a blood pressure check? If you use a random sampling system, such doubts can be minimised.

There are many different random sampling systems, but one simple method is to use a **random number table** (these can be purchased or downloaded) or a computer program to produce a **random number list** to select the sample. Free web-based resources can generate a random number list. For example, if you want a random sample of 50 from a population of 300, you could list all 300 subjects and assign a number to each. Then use the numbers on the random number list, which match the numbers you have assigned. This produces a simple random sample. Generating 50 random numbers from 300 produces a list like the one shown in Table 3.1.

Multi-stage sampling can also be used. For example, in a study of university students in the UK, it would be difficult to obtain a complete list of all students. Even if such a list were available, the sheer number of students would be difficult to manage. To overcome this problem, multi-stage sampling could involve first selecting a simple random sample of all UK universities (first stage), and then a simple random sample of student names could be drawn from each selected university (second stage). This approach saves time, as it avoids the need to study every university. Additional stages can be added to multi-stage sampling. For example, after randomly selecting the universities (first stage), a simple random sample of each university's faculties could be taken (second stage), and then a simple random sample of students within each faculty (third stage). Although multi-stage sampling can provide better focus and save resources, it will yield less precise results than would be obtained by taking a simple random sample from a complete list of all UK university students.

TABLE 3.1 Random number list showing 50 random numbers

8	12	14	22	24	27	33	37	49
55	67	78	79	93	95	98	104	108
113	116	125	128	129	133	138	143	158
163	167	169	171	173	176	184	193	203
212	218	219	221	224	225	230	232	249
264	272	273	283	285				

Cluster sampling is similar to multi-stage sampling, except that **all** of the subjects in the final-stage sample are investigated. In the three-stage example just described, the randomly selected faculties would be regarded as **clusters**, and all students within these faculties would be studied.

It can be useful to employ **stratified sampling** to randomly select subjects from different strata or groups. Imagine a study designed to examine possible variations in healthcare between Asian and non-Asian patients. A random sample of patients on a list would almost certainly produce very few Asian patients, as most localities have a lower proportion of Asian residents. In such a case, we could stratify our sample by dividing patients into Asian and non-Asian subjects, and then take a random sample of the same size for each.

A less random but nevertheless useful approach is to use a **systematic sampling** scheme. In this method, a number is assigned to every record, and then every *n*th record is selected from a list. For example, if you want to systematically select 50 of your 300 patients with angina, the procedure would be as follows:

1. Obtain a list of all 300 patients with angina (this is your sampling frame).
2. As 300/50 = 6, you will be taking every sixth patient.
3. Choose a number randomly between 1 and 6 as a starting point.
4. Take every sixth patient thereafter (e.g. if your starting point is 4, you will take patient numbers 4, 10, 16, 22, 28, 34, etc.).

By doing this, you are using the list rather than your own judgement to select the patients. Look at the list carefully before you start selecting. For example, choosing every tenth patient in a list of married couples may well result in every selected person being male or every selected person being female (Donaldson & Scally, 2009).

For randomised controlled trials (*see* Chapter 31), random number tables can also be used to allocate patients to treatment groups. For example, the first number in the table can be allocated to the first patient, the second number to the second patient and so on. Odd numbers may be allocated to treatment group A, and even numbers to treatment group B. Other methods include subjects being randomly allocated to treatment groups by opening sealed envelopes containing details of the treatment category.

CHAPTER 4

Presenting data

A variety of graph styles can be used to present data. The most commonly used types of graph are pie charts, bar diagrams, histograms and scattergrams.

The purpose of using a graph is to tell others about a set of data **quickly**, allowing them to grasp the important characteristics of the data. In other words, graphs are visual aids to rapid understanding. It is therefore important to make graphs as simple and easy to understand as possible. The use of 'three-dimensional' and other special effects can detract from easy and accurate understanding. Such approaches should therefore be avoided altogether, or used with great care. Also, omitting '0' from a scale can make the graph misleading. Some examples of graphs follow.

The graph in Figure 4.1 is known as a **pie chart**, because it depicts each category as a slice of pie, with the size of each slice varying according to its proportion of the whole pie. This can be useful for comparing individual categories with the total. The pie chart in Figure 4.1 shows the distribution of different visual impairments in Swiss pathologists. It is easy to see that myopia (nearsightedness) was recorded most frequently, and that 8.6% of those with a visual impairment had hyperopia (farsightedness).

Figure 4.2 shows an example of a **bar diagram**. In this example, the size of each block represents the frequency recorded for the category concerned. Bar diagrams are useful for comparing one category with others. In the bar diagram shown in Figure 4.2, we can see the percentage of musculoskeletal problems recorded in Swiss pathologists. It is clear that the percentage of neck problems was nearly three times higher than hand/arm problems.

The graph shown in Figure 4.3 is called a **histogram**. Histograms are bar diagrams, where the areas (i.e. height **and** width) of the bars are proportional to the frequencies in each group. These are especially useful for frequency distributions of grouped data (e.g. age groups, grouped heights, grouped blood measurements). For example, if you use age groups of equal range (e.g. 21–30, 31–40, 41–50 years, etc.), then the width of each bar is equal, and if the 21–30 years age group has a frequency of 30, while the 31–40 years age group has a frequency of 60, then the former group is exactly half the

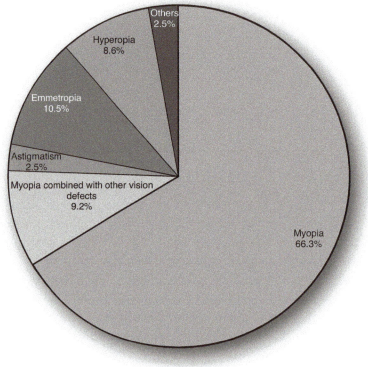

FIGURE 4.1 Distribution of different visual impairments among Swiss pathologists. Source: Adapted from Fritzsche *et al.* (2012).

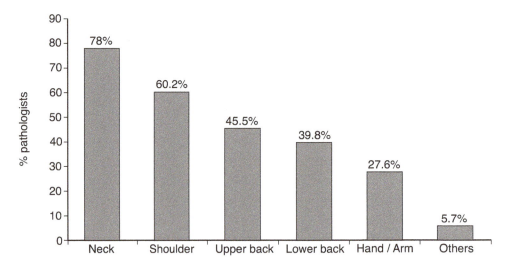

FIGURE 4.2 Location of musculoskeletal problems in Swiss pathologists. Source: Adapted from Fritzsche *et al.* (2012).

height of the latter. The histogram in Figure 4.3 shows the frequency distribution of patients presenting with myelodysplastic syndrome in a given period, with the patients grouped into 5-year blocks.

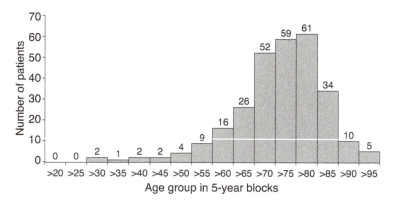

FIGURE 4.3 Age distribution of patients presenting with myelodysplastic syndrome in Bournemouth 1981–90. Adapted from Oscier (1997).

An example of a **scatterplot** is shown in Figure 4.4. In a scatterplot, two measurements (also called **variables**) are each plotted on separate axes. The variable on the (horizontal) x-**axis** is usually called the **independent variable**, and the variable on the (vertical) y-**axis** is usually called the **dependent variable**. You can usually tell which variable is dependent on the other by considering which variable could have been caused by which other variable. In Figure 4.4, the weight of an adult patient **can** depend on (or be caused by) his or her height, whereas height **cannot** be dependent on (or caused by) weight. Scatterplots are discussed further in Chapter 18.

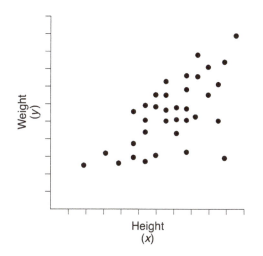

FIGURE 4.4 Example of a scatterplot.

CHAPTER 5

Frequencies, percentages, proportions and rates

Suppose we ask a sample of 30 teenagers each to tell us how old they are. The list of their ages is shown in Table 5.1:

TABLE 5.1 List of ages from a sample of teenagers

15	14	16	15	17	14	16	17	14	18
19	16	17	14	13	15	14	16	16	19
19	18	14	17	14	16	15	17	15	17

This is all very well, but when the data are presented in this way, it is difficult to make sense of them quickly. For example, how many of the teenagers are old enough to drive? How many of them are old enough to purchase alcohol legally? Are there more 15-year-olds than 16-year-olds in this group? From the listing shown, it is difficult to answer these questions. Individual ages need to be picked out and counted up **every time** we want to answer such a question.

A summary of the data can make things easier. What if we count up how often each individual age is recorded, and write this down? Then we can look at the count each time we need to know something about these ages. In Table 5.2, the ages are sorted into numerical order, and the number of times each age is recorded is written at the side.

It is now easy to see how often each age occurs. We can quickly tell that 11 teenagers are old enough to drive (the legal age is 17 years in the UK), 5 can legally purchase alcohol (the legal age is 18 years in the UK) and there are more 16-year-olds ($n = 6$) than 15-year-olds ($n = 5$).

The number of times that something occurs is known as its **frequency**. For example, the frequency of 14-year-olds in our sample is 7, and the frequency of 18-year-olds is 2. Table 5.2 shows the ages and their frequencies, and is called a **frequency distribution**. It shows how the ages are distributed in this sample.

TABLE 5.2 Frequency distribution of age

Age (years)	Number of times recorded
13	1
14	7
15	5
16	6
17	6
18	2
19	3

In the frequency distribution in Table 5.3, the frequencies are added up and **percentages** added (in this example, the percentages are rounded up to the nearest whole per cent). This is a common way of presenting a frequency distribution.

The percentages indicate the **proportion** of times that a particular age is recorded. Proportions can be expressed as decimals or multiplied by 100 and expressed as percentages.

For example, if 15 out of 30 teenagers are aged 18 years, then the proportion is **0.50** (15/30 = 0.50) or the percentage is **50%** (0.50 × 100 = 50).

Note that in statistics, we normally use the symbol '/' for division, instead of '÷'.

If 20 of the teenagers are aged 18 years, then the proportion is **0.67** (20/30 = 0.666 or **0.67 to two decimal places**) or **67%** (0.67 × 100 = 67).

TABLE 5.3 Frequency distribution of age, also showing totals and percentages

Age	Frequency	%
13	1	3
14	7	23
15	5	17
16	6	20
17	6	20
18	2	7
19	3	10
Total	30	100

In Table 5.3, 5 of the 30 teenagers are aged 15 years. The proportion is **0.17** (5/30 = 0.1666 **or 0.17 to two decimal places**), and the percentage is **17%** (0.17 × 100 = 17).

In these calculations, we have sometimes rounded numbers to two **decimal places**. For example, if we use a calculator to work out 20/30, it will probably display '0.6666666' – it has displayed seven numbers after the decimal point. This is called 'displaying to seven decimal places'. To show this as three decimal places, we round the third digit after the decimal point **up** to the nearest whole number. Thus when displaying 0.6666666 to three decimal places, 0.667 is nearer to the real value than is 0.666. In other words, if the last digit is 5 or more, we round **up** to the next whole number. If we want to round 1.222 to two decimal places, 1.22 is nearer to the true value than 1.23. So if the last digit is 4 or less, we round **down** to the nearest number.

Proportions or percentages are more useful than frequencies when we want to compare numbers of events in two or more groups of **unequal size**. For example, suppose that we want to compare the number of industrial accidents in the work forces of two different companies. In company A, there have been 37 accidents among a total of 267 workers. In company B, 45 accidents have occurred among a total of 385 workers. At which company are workers more likely to have an accident? On the face of it, company B has experienced more accidents, but it also employs more workers. Unless you are very good at mental arithmetic, it is difficult to answer the question. Let us work it out using proportions:

- company A had 37 accidents among 267 workers – the proportion of accidents is 0.139 (37/267)
- company B had 45 accidents among 385 workers – the proportion of accidents is 0.117 (45/385).

Therefore even though company A's workforce had fewer accidents, it is statistically the more dangerous place to work, as it had a higher proportion of accidents. When we use proportions to describe the number of events, they can be called **rates**. In this example, therefore, the **accident rate** in company A is 0.139 (or 13.9%) and that in company B is 0.117 (or 11.7%).

CHAPTER 6

Types of data

At this stage, it is worth mentioning the need to recognise different types of data. For example, we could ask people to give us information about how old they are in one of two ways. We could ask them to tell us how old they are in whole years (i.e. their age last birthday). Alternatively, we could ask them to tell us to which of several specified age bands they belong (e.g. 20–24, 25–29, 30–34 years, etc.). Although these two methods tell us about the age of the respondents, hopefully you can see that the two types of data are not the same!

Data can be classified as either **categorical** or **numerical**.

CATEGORICAL DATA

This refers to data that are arranged into separate categories. Categorical data are also called **qualitative** data.

If there are only two possible categories (e.g. yes/no, female or male), the data are said to be **dichotomous**. If there are more possible categories (e.g. a range of several age groups or ethnic minority groups), the data may be described as **nominal**.

Categories can sometimes be placed in order. In this case they are called **ordinal data**. For example, a questionnaire may ask respondents how happy they are with the quality of catering in hospital, the choices may be very happy, quite happy, unhappy or very unhappy. Other examples of ordinal data include positions in hospital league tables, and tumour stages. Because the data are arranged both in categories **and** in order, ordinal data provide more information than categories alone.

NUMERICAL DATA

For this type of data, numbers are used instead of categories. Numerical data are also called **quantitative** data.

There are three levels (scales) of numerical data. These are presented in order according to how much information they contain.

In **discrete** data, all values are clearly separate from each other. Although numbers are used, they can only have a certain range of values. For example, age last birthday is usually given as a whole number (e.g. 22 or 35, rather than 22.45 or 35.6, etc.). Other examples of discrete data include the number of operations performed in 1 year, or the number of newly diagnosed asthma cases in 1 month. It is usually acceptable to analyse discrete data as if they were continuous. For example, it is reasonable to calculate the mean number (*see* Chapter 7) of total knee replacement operations that are performed in a year.

The next two scales are regarded as **continuous** – each value can have any number of values in between, depending on the accuracy of measurement (for example, there can be many smaller values in between a height of 2 m and a height of 3 m, e.g. 2.2 or 2.23 or 2.23978675). Continuous data can also be converted into categorical or discrete data. For example, a list of heights can be converted into grouped categories, and temperature values in degrees centigrade (measured to one or more decimal places) can each be converted to the nearest whole degree centigrade.

In **interval** data, values are separated by **equally spaced** intervals (e.g. weight, height, minutes, degrees centigrade). Thus the difference (or interval) between 5 kg and 10 kg, for example, is exactly the same as that between 20 kg and 25 kg. As interval data allow us to tell the precise interval between any one value and another, they give more information than discrete data. Interval data can also be converted into categorical or discrete data. For example, a list of temperature measurements in degrees centigrade can be placed in ordered categories or grouped into dichotomous categories of 'afebrile' (oral temperature below 37°C) or 'febrile' (oral temperature of 37°C or more).

Ratio data are similar to interval scales, but refer to the ratio of two measurements and also have a true zero. Thus weight in kilograms is an example of ratio data (20 kg is twice as heavy as 10 kg, and it is theoretically possible for something to weigh 0 kg). However, degrees centigrade cannot be considered to be a ratio scale (20°C is not, in any meaningful way, twice as warm as 10°C, and the degrees centigrade scale extends below 0°C). Ratio data are also interval data.

Sometimes people get different types of data confused – with alarming results. The following is a real example (although the numbers have been changed to guarantee anonymity). As part of a study, a researcher asks a group of 70 pregnant women to state which of a range of age groups they belong to. These are entered into a table as shown in Table 6.1.

TABLE 6.1 Table of age groups

Title given to age group	1	2	3	4	5	6	7
Age group (years)	≤16	17–21	22–26	27–31	32–36	37–41	≥42
Frequency	1	5	18	24	13	7	2

The researcher wants to enter the data into a computerised analysis program, and to ensure ease of data entry, he decides to give each group a numerical title (so that, when entering the data, he can simply press '3' for someone who is in the '22–26' years age group, for example). Unfortunately, he does not notice that the program assumes that the numerical titles represent continuous data. It therefore treats the age groups as if they were actual ages, rather than categories. Being busy with other matters, the researcher does not notice this in the program's data analysis output. In his report, he states that the mean age of the pregnant women is 4.03 years! Of course, the most frequently recorded age group (27–31 years), also called the mode (*see* Chapter 7), is the correct measure for these data. Treating categorical data as if they were continuous can thus produce very misleading results and is therefore dangerous. Clearly, great care needs to be taken to ensure that data are collected and analysed correctly.

Mean, median and mode

Means, medians and modes are methods of measuring the **central tendency** of a group of values – that is, the tendency for values in a group to gather around a central or 'average' value which is typical of the group.

MEAN

It can be very useful to summarise a group of numerical values by finding their **average** value. The mean gives a rough idea of the size of the values that you are dealing with, without having to look at every one of them. The mean (or to use its proper name, the **arithmetic mean**) is another term for the **average**.

Consider the $HbA1_c$ (the percentage of glycosylated haemoglobin circulating in the blood) values for patients with diabetes, shown in the frequency distribution in Figure 7.1. It also shows the median and mode, which are discussed later in this chapter.

The formula for calculating the mean is:

$\Sigma x/n$
Add up (Σ) all of the values (x) and divide by the number of values observed (n).

To calculate a mean:

1. add up every value in your group (call this result A)
2. count how many values are observed in the group (call this result B)
3. divide result A by result B.

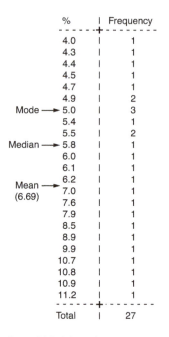

```
                    %      | Frequency
              - - - - -+- - - - - - - -
                   4.0    |     1
                   4.3    |     1
                   4.4    |     1
                   4.5    |     1
                   4.7    |     1
                   4.9    |     2
       Mode ─── 5.0       |     3
                   5.4    |     1
                   5.5    |     2
     Median ─── 5.8       |     1
                   6.0    |     1
                   6.1    |     1
                   6.2    |     1
       Mean ───
       (6.69)      7.0    |     1
                   7.6    |     1
                   7.9    |     1
                   8.5    |     1
                   8.9    |     1
                   9.9    |     1
                  10.7    |     1
                  10.8    |     1
                  10.9    |     1
                  11.2    |     1
              - - - - -+- - - - - - - -
                  Total   |    27
```

FIGURE 7.1 Frequency distribution of HbA1$_c$ values.

In the example in Figure 7.1:

1. the sum of all of the HbA1$_c$ values listed = 180.6
2. the number of values observed = 27
3. 180.6/27 = 6.69 (or 6.7 if we use one decimal place).

The mean is usually represented by $\bar{x}$ (called **x-bar**) for samples, and μ (called **mu**) for populations.

Remember that, when writing the mean, it is good practice to refer to the **unit** measured. In this case, it is a **HbA1$_c$ value** of 6.7%.

Note that many calculators will work out the mean in a single process, without having to go through the steps outlined here.

The mean can be misleading if there are any **extreme** values in a group of numbers. For example, the mean of the group 1, 2, 3, 2, 4, 5, 19 is 5.1. The value 19 is an extreme value, as it is far higher than any of the other numbers in the group. Since only one of the values in the group is actually 5.1 or greater, the mean is not representative of the group. In this case, the **median** may provide a better representation.

MEDIAN

This is the middle value of an ordered sample of numerical values. To calculate the median:

1. arrange all of the recorded values in order of size
2. find the middle value.

If we arrange the following numbers in numerical order, we obtain:

$$1, 2, 2, \mathbf{3}, 4, 5, 19.$$

The median is **3**.

In this example, the median is much more representative of the group than the mean (5.1). Extreme values do not affect the median, and the median value is usually typical of the data.

If there is an even number of values, use the mean of the two middle values:

$$19, 24, \mathbf{26}, \mathbf{30}, 31, 34.$$

The median is (26 + 30)/2 = 28.

The median $HbA1_c$ value in Figure 7.1 is **5.8** – there are 13 values below and 13 values above it.

MODE

The **mode** is the value which occurs most often in a group. This can be a group of either numbers or categories.

In Figure 7.1, the $HbA1_c$ value **5.0** is recorded more often than any other value (three times in all), and so it is the mode of that group.

For example, if you want to know the most frequently used health promotion clinic (e.g. 'smoking cessation', 'weight loss', 'well woman', 'well man', etc.) at a primary care surgery, count up the attendance at each clinic over a specific period, and find the one with the highest attendance.

If there are two modes in a group of numbers, the group is described as **bimodal**. The mode is easy to determine, and requires no calculation. It is usually typical of the data used. Because the mode only records the most popular value, the others are not taken into account. The mode is therefore not affected by extreme values.

The mode can be used for categorical data where the mean and median are not appropriate (e.g. as in the example shown in Table 6.1).

CHAPTER 8

Centiles

Although the median is the middle value in a group of ordered numbers, it provides no information about the range of values, or how the values are grouped around the median. The **range** uses only the highest and lowest values, which may be extreme values. As we have already found when discussing the mean, extreme values may provide a misleading representation of the central tendency of the group. One approach is to effectively ignore a percentage of values at each end of the group, and to concentrate on the central area, where the majority of values are likely to lie.

Centiles allow us to describe the central range of a group of numbers. They are often expressed as the 25th and 75th centiles, although it is possible to calculate centiles of any value (e.g. 3rd and 97th centiles). Centiles are also referred to as **percentiles**.

The **25th centile** is also called the **first quartile**. It is the point which separates the **lower** quarter of the numbers in a group, in the same way as the median separates the **upper** half. The **50th centile** is also called the **second quartile**, and is equivalent to the median. The **75th centile** is also called the **third quartile**, and is the point that separates the upper quarter of the numbers.

The **interquartile range** is the distance between the 25th and 75th centiles, and is calculated by simply subtracting the 25th centile from the 75th centile. It provides an indication of how much variation (or spread) there is between the first and third quartiles. It ignores the values below the first quartile and above the third quartile.

For example, suppose that a group of patients has the following cholesterol values (in mmol/L):

3.5, 3.5, 3.6, **3.7**, 4.0, 4.1, 4.3, **4.5**, 4.7, 4.8, 5.2, **5.7**, 6.1, 6.3, 6.3

The 25th centile is **3.7**. The 50th centile (median) is **4.5**. The 75th centile is **5.7**. The interquartile range is: (5.7 − 3.7) = **2.0**.

This means that there is a variation of 2.0 mmol/L between the first and third quartiles, and a range of 3.5–6.3 mmol/L. A second group of patients may have an interquartile range of 0.9 mmol/L, indicating less variation. Even if the first and last values in the second group are very extreme (e.g. 3.0 and 9.0, respectively), these will not affect the interquartile range, which concentrates on the central area of values.

CHAPTER 9

Standard deviation

We have seen that the interquartile range indicates the variation of data where the median is the measure of central tendency. Standard deviation is used where this measure is the **mean**. It indicates the difference between a group of values and their mean, taking **all** of the data into account. Although this means that it may be influenced by extreme values, the standard deviation plays an important role in many tests of statistical significance (which will be described in later chapters). The larger the standard deviation, the more the values differ from the mean, and therefore the more widely they are spread out.

For example, one small group of patients in a particular outpatient clinic may wait for a mean time of 11 minutes to be seen by a doctor, and the standard deviation from the mean for this group is 5.701. Individual waiting times vary widely – from 7 minutes up to 21 minutes. There is wide variation between these waiting times, and they are quite widely spread out from their mean. These waiting times are therefore **heterogeneous** or dissimilar.

On another day, another group of patients from the same clinic may also have a mean waiting time of 11 minutes, but their standard deviation is 0.707. This is much less than the first group's standard deviation of 5.701. Looking at this group's actual waiting times, it can be seen that they only vary from 10 to 12 minutes. Waiting times for the second group are more **homogeneous** – that is, the data are more similar to each other. They are less widely spread out around their mean than the first group.

Let us look at the actual waiting times recorded for each group, as shown in Table 9.1.

You can see that the data in group 1 are much more spread out than those in group 2. This difference in standard deviations can be explained by the fact that, although most patients in group 1 waited a very short time, one patient had to wait for a long time (21 minutes). Although this one 'outlier' waiting time is not representative of the whole group, it has a large effect on the overall results, and it strongly affects the mean and standard deviation. Several patients from group 2 actually waited longer than group 1 patients, although the difference between the waiting times in group 2 is very slight.

TABLE 9.1 Waiting times and standard deviation for each patient group

Group	Time 1	Time 2	Time 3	Time 4	Time 5	Mean	Standard deviation
1	10	7	8	9	21	11	5.701
2	11	11	10	11	12	11	0.707

Although the abbreviations **SD** or **s.d.** are used to represent standard deviation generally, s is used to represent standard deviation for **samples**, and σ is used to represent standard deviation for **populations**.

The most usual formula for standard deviation is as follows:

$$\sqrt{\Sigma(x-\bar{x})^2/(n-1)}$$

where x = individual value, $\bar{x}$ = sample mean and n = number of values.

The equation is only suitable for a sample (or **population estimate**). This will usually be the case, since we rarely know the true population value (which in this case is the mean).

The following steps are used to work out a standard deviation.

1. Find the mean of the group.
2. Subtract this from every value in the group individually – this shows the deviation from the mean, for every value.
3. Work out the square (x^2) of every deviation (that is, multiply each deviation by itself, e.g. $5^2 = 5 \times 5 = 25$) – this produces a squared deviation for every value.
4. Add up all of the squared deviations.
5. Add up the number of observed values, and subtract 1.
6. Divide the sum of squared deviations by this number, to produce the **sample variance**.
7. Work out the square root of the variance.

If you have to work out a standard deviation by hand, it is helpful to use a grid like the one shown in Table 9.2. We can use this to work out the standard deviation of the data for group 1 from Table 9.1.

TABLE 9.2 Grid showing preliminary calculations for standard deviation

Value number	Time (a)	Mean time (b)	Deviation from the mean (a − b)	Squared deviation (a–b)²
1	10	11	−1	1
2	7	11	−4	16
3	8	11	−3	9
4	9	11	−2	4
5	21	11	10	100
				Total = 130

1. We already know the mean is 11 (*see* previous page).
2. Subtract each time value from the mean. Note each result in the 'Deviation from the mean' column.
3. Multiply each deviation by itself, and write each result in the 'Squared deviation' column (e.g. $-4^2 = -4 \times -4 = 16$) (note that multiplying **minus** numbers produces **positive** ones).
4. Adding all of the squared deviations (1 + 16 + 9 + 4 + 100) gives a value of 130.
5. There are five separate values in the group. Subtract 1, and you get 4.
6. Divide the sum of squared deviations by 4, to produce the variance (130/4 = 32.5).
7. Use a calculator to determine the square root of the variance (32.5) – that $\sqrt{32.5}$ = **5.701**.

Of course, calculating standard deviation by hand like this is not practical if you have a large number of values. Moreover, the mean is unlikely to be a whole number as it is in the example here. Calculators and computer programs are an invaluable aid to this process, and are readily available.

Other uses of standard deviation are discussed under normal distribution (*see* Chapter 11).

CHAPTER 10

Standard error

Standard error (or **s.e.**) is another term for the standard deviation of a **sampling distribution** (or frequency distribution of samples), rather than just a sample. You may remember from Chapter 2 that a value found from one sample may be different to that from another sample – this is called **sampling variation**. For example, if we took a large number of samples of a particular size from a population and recorded the mean for each sample, we could calculate the standard deviation of all their means – this is called the **standard error**. Because it is based on a very large number of (theoretical) samples, it should be more precise and therefore smaller than the standard deviation.

Standard error is used in a range of applications, including **hypothesis testing** and the calculation of **confidence intervals** (which are discussed in later chapters).

The most frequently used calculations are described as follows:

COMPARING A SAMPLE MEAN WITH A POPULATION MEAN (FOR LARGE SAMPLES)

$$\text{s.e.} = s/\sqrt{n}$$

Divide the standard deviation (s) by the square root of the number of values (n) in the sample.

To calculate the standard error, follow the steps listed below.

1. Calculate the standard deviation of the sample mean.
2. Count the number of observed values.
3. Find the square root of this sum.
4. Divide the standard deviation by this number.

Using the table of HbA1$_c$ values in Figure 7.1 in Chapter 7, we can calculate the standard error as follows:

1. The standard deviation is 2.322 (not shown in Chapter 7).
2. The number of observed values = 27.
3. The square root of 27 = 5.196.
4. Divide the standard deviation (2.322) by 5.196 = **0.447**.

You can see that the standard error is very much smaller than the standard deviation.

COMPARING TWO SAMPLE MEANS (FOR LARGE SAMPLES)

$$\text{s.e.} = \sqrt{\frac{s_1^2 + s_2^2}{n_1 + n_2}}$$

where: s_1 = standard deviation for sample 1, s_2 = standard deviation for sample 2, n_1 = sample size 1 and n_2 = sample size 2.

Let us work through the stages of this formula.

1. Square the first sample standard deviation (s_1).
2. Divide it by the first sample size (n_1) – note the result, and call it 'result 1'.
3. Square the second sample standard deviation (s_2).
4. Divide it by the second sample size (n_2) – note this result, and call it 'result 2'.
5. Add results 1 and 2.
6. Find the square root of this number – this is the standard error.

SINGLE PROPORTION (FOR LARGE SAMPLES)

$$\text{s.e.} = \sqrt{\frac{p(1-p)}{n}}$$

where p = proportion and n = sample size.

There are different formulae for calculating standard error in other situations (e.g. for comparing proportions in two independent groups, where the sample size is large), and these are covered by several other texts.

Standard error formulae for **small** samples are presented in Chapter 15.

CHAPTER 11

Normal distribution

If we take a large sample of men or women, measure their heights and plot them on a frequency distribution, the distribution will almost certainly obtain a symmetrical bell-shaped pattern that looks something like the one shown in Figure 11.1.

This is known as the **normal distribution** (also called the Gaussian distribution). The least frequently recorded heights lie at the two extremes of the curve. It can be seen that very few women are **extremely** short or **extremely** tall. An outline of the normal distribution curve is drawn around the frequency distribution, and is a reasonably good fit to the shape of the distribution. With a larger sample size, the pattern of the frequency distribution will usually follow this shape more closely.

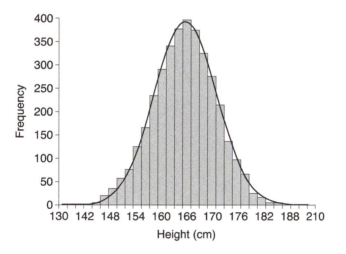

FIGURE 11.1 Distribution of a sample of values of women's heights.

In practice, many biological measurements follow this pattern, making it possible to use the normal distribution to describe many features of a population.

It must be emphasised that some measurements do not follow the symmetrical shape of the normal distribution, and can be **positively skewed** or **negatively skewed**. For example, more of the populations of developed Western countries are becoming obese. If a large sample of such a population's weights was to be plotted on a graph similar to that in Figure 11.1, there would be an excess of heavier weights which might form a similar shape to the 'negatively skewed' example in Figure 11.2. The distribution will therefore not fit the symmetrical pattern of the normal distribution. You can tell whether the skew is positive or negative by looking at the shape of the plotted data, as shown in Figure 11.2.

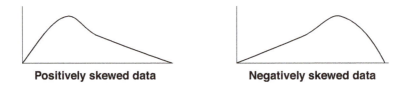

FIGURE 11.2 Examples of positive and negative skew.

Furthermore, the shape may be symmetrical but different to the normal distribution.

The normal distribution is shown in Figure 11.3. You can see that it is split into two equal and identically shaped halves by the mean. The standard deviation indicates the size of the spread of the data. It can also help us to determine how likely it is that a given value will be observed in the population being studied. We know this because the proportion of the population that is covered by any number of standard deviations can be calculated.

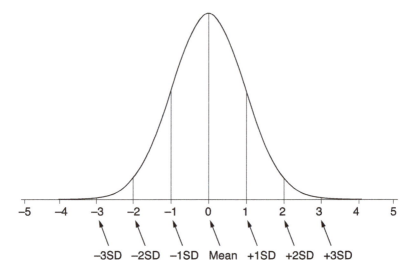

FIGURE 11.3 The normal distribution.

For example:

- **68.27%** of all values lie within plus or minus (±) one standard deviation (either one standard deviation below the mean or one standard deviation above it)
- **95.45%** of all values lie within ± two standard deviations of the mean
- **99.73%** of all values lie within ± three standard deviations of the mean.

It is useful to know that 95% of all values lie within 1.96 standard deviations, and 99% of all values lie within 2.58 standard deviations.

The proportions of values **below** and **above** a specified value (e.g. the mean) can be calculated, and are known as **tails**. We shall discuss these in Chapter 14.

It is possible to calculate the probability that a value in any particular range will occur. The normal distribution is useful in a number of applications, including confidence intervals (*see* Chapter 12) and hypothesis testing (*see* Chapter 14).

As well as the normal distribution, a number of other distributions are important, including the following:

- the *t*-**distribution** – for small samples (usually below 30) (*see* Chapter 15 on *t*-tests)
- the **binomial distribution** – for dichotomous data (e.g. result can only be 0 or 1; yes or no)
- the **Poisson distribution** – for rare events that occur randomly in a large population.

The *t*- and binomial distributions resemble the normal distribution when large samples are used.

CHAPTER 12

Confidence intervals

This interval has been constructed from the random sample data using a procedure such that, if we took many such samples and constructed a confidence interval for each, then 95% of the varying intervals would contain the population mean (a fixed, but unknown value).

Although we can calculate a sample mean, we never know **exactly** where the population mean is. Confidence intervals are used to estimate how far away the population mean is likely to be, with a given degree of certainty. This technique is called **estimation**, and the term 'confidence interval' is often abbreviated to **c.i.** or **CI**. Conventionally, 95% confidence intervals are used, although they can be calculated for 99% or any other value.

Figure 12.1 shows diastolic blood pressure measurements taken from a sample of 92 patients with diabetes. The mean diastolic blood pressure is 82.696 mmHg, with a standard error of 1.116. A 95% confidence interval will indicate a range **above and below** 82.696 mmHg in which the population mean will lie, with a 95% degree of certainty. In other words, a '95% confidence interval' is the interval which will include the **true** population value in 95% of cases.

The formula for calculating a 95% confidence interval for a sample mean (large samples) is:

$$\bar{x} \pm (1.96 \times \text{s.e.})$$

where $\bar{x}$ = sample mean and s.e. = standard error.

This formula is suitable for samples of around 30 or larger, where data are on the interval or ratio scale, and are normally distributed.

Note that numbers in this section are calculated to three decimal places.

To calculate a 95% confidence interval (large samples), follow the steps listed next.

```
Diastolic        |  Frequency
blood pressure   |
(mmHg)           |
---------+----------
   50    |     1
   60    |     1
   64    |     1
   66    |     1
   70    |    15
   72    |     1
   78    |     2       Mean = 82.696
   80    |    33       Sample size (n) = 92
   84    |     3       Standard deviation = 10.701
   85    |     1       Standard error = 1.116
   88    |     2
   90    |    14
   93    |     1
   94    |     1
   95    |     4
  100    |    10
  110    |     1
---------+--------
  Total  |    92
```

FIGURE 12.1 Frequency distribution of diastolic blood pressure in a sample of patients with diabetes. Source: Unpublished data from Stewart and Rao (2000).

1. Calculate the sample mean, the standard deviation and hence the standard error (s.e.).
2. Multiply the s.e. by 1.96, and note this result (call it **result 1**).
3. Add **result 1** to the sample mean, and note this sum (call it *sum a*).
4. Take **result 1** away from the sample mean, and note this sum (call it *sum b*).
5. The confidence interval is written as:

   95% c.i. = (sample mean) ((*sum a*) → (*sum b*)).

Let us work through this using the diastolic blood pressure readings in Figure 12.1.

1. The sample mean is 82.696; the standard error (s.e.) is 1.116 (remember that the standard error is calculated as $10.701/\sqrt{92}$.
2. s.e. × 1.96 = 1.116 × 1.96 = 2.187.
3. 82.696 + 2.187 = 84.883.
4. 82.696–2.187 = 80.509.
5. **95% c.i. is 82.696 (80.509 → 84.883).**

In the example, although the sample mean is 82.696, there is a 95% degree of certainty that the **population** mean lies between 80.509 and 84.883. In this case, the range is not particularly wide, indicating that the population mean is unlikely to be far away.

It should therefore be reasonably representative of patients with diabetes, so long as the sample was randomly selected. Increasing the sample size will usually result in a narrower confidence interval.

To calculate a 99% confidence interval, use **2.58** instead of 1.96 (this is the number of standard deviations which contain 99% of all the values of the normal distribution). Although a 99% confidence interval will give greater certainty, the intervals will be wider.

In the example here, we have calculated a confidence interval for a single mean, based on a fairly large sample. Confidence intervals can be calculated for other circumstances, some of which are listed as follows:

- 95% c.i. for difference between two sample means – **large samples**:

$$(\overline{x}_1 - \overline{x}_2) \pm (1.96 \times \text{s.e.})$$

  (*see* s.e. formula for comparing two sample means (large samples) in Chapter 10)

- 95% c.i. for a single proportion (p) – **large samples**:

$$p \pm (1.96 \times \text{s.e.})$$

  (*see* s.e. formula for single proportion (large samples) in Chapter 10).

There are different formulae for calculating confidence intervals and standard error in other situations (e.g. for comparing proportions in two independent groups, where the sample size is large), and these are covered by several other texts.

- For **small samples**:

$$\overline{x} \pm t \times \text{s.e.}$$

  (also *see* Chapter 15 on t-tests).

CHAPTER 13

Probability

Probability is a mathematical technique for predicting outcomes. It predicts how likely it is that specific events will occur.

Probability is measured on a scale from 0 to 1.0 as shown in Figure 13.1.

For example, when one tosses a coin, there is a 50% chance of obtaining a head. Note that probabilities are usually expressed in **decimal** format – 50% becomes 0.5, 10% becomes 0.1 and 5% becomes 0.05. The probability of obtaining a head when a coin is tossed is therefore 0.5.

A probability can **never** be more than 1.0, nor can it be negative.

There is a range of methods for calculating probability for different situations.

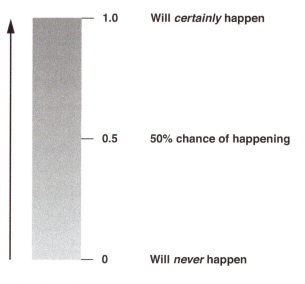

FIGURE 13.1 The scale of probability.

TO CALCULATE THE PROBABILITY (*P*) OF A *SINGLE EVENT* (A) HAPPENING

For example, to find the probability of throwing a six on a die:

$$\text{formula:} \quad P(A) = \frac{\text{the number of possible events}}{\text{the number of possible equally likely outcomes}}$$

$$P(A) = \frac{\text{the number of sixes on the die}}{\text{the number of sides on the die}}$$

$$= \frac{1}{6} = \mathbf{0.1667} \text{ (or 16.67\%)}$$

TO CALCULATE THE PROBABILITY OF EVENT (A) *AND* EVENT (B) HAPPENING (INDEPENDENT EVENTS)

For example, if you have two identical packs of cards (pack A and pack B), what is the probability of drawing the ace of spades from **both** packs?

Formula: $P(A) \times P(B)$
$P(\text{pack A}) = 1$ card, from a pack of 52 cards = 1/52 = 0.0192
$P(\text{pack B}) = 1$ card, from a pack of 52 cards = 1/52 = 0.0192
$P(A) \times P(B) = 0.0192 \times 0.0192 = \mathbf{0.00037}$

This is called the **rule of multiplication**.

In the example, events A and B are **independent** of each other. This means that one event happens regardless of the other, and its outcome is not related to the other.

Sometimes probabilities are **conditional**, which means that one probability relies on another having already happened.

TO CALCULATE THE PROBABILITY OF EVENT (A) *AND* EVENT (B) HAPPENING (CONDITIONAL EVENTS)

What is the probability of drawing the ace of spades **and** the queen of clubs consecutively from a single pack of cards?

Formula: $P(A) \times P(B \mid A)$

where $(B \mid A)$ means

[**B given that** A has happened]

We already know that the probability of drawing the ace of spades from a pack of 52 cards is 1/52 = 0.0192, so $P(A) = 0.0192$.

The chances of now drawing the queen of clubs are a little higher, because one less card is left in the pack, so the probability $P(B \mid A)$ is now 1/51 = 0.0196.

$$P(A) \times P(B \mid A) = (1/52) \times (1/51) = 0.0192 \times 0.0196 = 0.0004$$

Probabilities can be **mutually exclusive**. This means that one event prevents another event from happening. For example, throwing a die once will result in either a one, **or** a two, **or** a three, **or** a four, **or** a five, **or** a six – but only **one** number can be obtained. Therefore throwing a five rules out any other number. In such cases, the rule of addition is used.

TO CALCULATE THE PROBABILITY OF *EITHER* EVENT (A) *OR* EVENT (B) HAPPENING (WHERE THE EVENTS ARE MUTUALLY EXCLUSIVE)

For example, what is the probability of throwing either a six or a five on a die?

Formula: $P(A) + P(B)$
$P(A) = 0.1667$
$P(B) = 0.1667$
$P(A) + P(B) = 0.1667 + 0.1667 = \mathbf{0.333}$ (or 33.3%)

This is called the **rule of addition** or the **additive rule**.

TO CALCULATE THE PROBABILITY OF *EITHER* EVENT (A) OR EVENT (B) HAPPENING (WHERE THE EVENTS ARE *NOT* MUTUALLY EXCLUSIVE)

Suppose that a local study finds that 90% of people aged over 60 years in Epitown suffer from at least one common cold during a 1-year period, and 20% suffer from heartburn at least once. What is the probability that any person over 60 years of age will suffer from **either** common cold **or** heartburn? We shall assume that common cold and heartburn occur independently of each other.

Using the rule of addition produces a probability of 0.9 + 0.2, which is equal to 1.1. This cannot be correct, since we already know that a probability can never be more than 1.0.

In this situation, we use a different formula:

$P(A) + P(B) - P$ (both)
$P(A) = 0.9$ (common cold)
$P(B) = 0.2$ (heartburn)
P (both) $= 0.9 \times 0.2 = 0.18$
(since we are assuming that they are independent).
So $P(A) + P(B) - P$(both) $= (0.9 + 0.2) - 0.18$
$\qquad\qquad\qquad\qquad\quad = 1.1 - 0.18$
$\qquad\qquad\qquad\qquad\quad = \mathbf{0.92}$ (or 92%)

In this example, then, there is a probability of 0.92 (or 92%) that any person aged over 60 years in Epitown will suffer from either common cold or heartburn during a 1-year period.

CHAPTER 14

Hypothesis tests and *P*-values

A **hypothesis** is an **unproved theory** that is formulated as a starting point for an investigation – for example, 'patients who take drug A will have better outcomes than those who take drug B' or 'drug A is better than drug B'. The hypothesis that 'drug A is better than drug B' is often written as H_1.

For every hypothesis there is a **null hypothesis**. In the scenarios mentioned, the null hypothesis is that 'the outcomes of patients taking drug A will be **the same as** those of patients who take drug B'. Scientific experiments tend to adopt a somewhat sceptical attitude, and normally use the null hypothesis to try to disprove the real hypothesis. The null hypothesis is often written as H_0.

If drug A proves to be significantly better than drug B, the null hypothesis (H_0) is rejected, and the **alternative hypothesis** (H_1) is accepted. Hypotheses are sometimes referred to as one-tailed or two-tailed. As described in Chapter 11, the normal distribution is split in half by the mean. The proportions of values **under** and **above** a specified value (e.g. two standard deviations more than the mean) can be calculated. These are known as **tails**. The term **one-tailed** refers to the distribution either under or above a specified value. The term **two-tailed** refers to the whole distribution, **both** under and above the specified value (e.g. either two standard deviations less or two standard deviations more). In a **two-tailed hypothesis**, we want to find out whether there will actually be a difference between the two treatments, but we do not state which way it will go (e.g. 'drug A will be better or worse than drug B'. In a **one-tailed hypothesis**, we are interested in the direction of any difference (e.g. 'drug A is **better** than drug B'). The two-tailed hypothesis is usually more appropriate.

The problem is how much better does the difference or **size of effect** need to be in order to reach the level of statistical **significance**? In practice, we assess **the probability that the effect we found (or a more extreme effect) would have occurred if the null hypothesis were true**. If the probability is low, it follows that the effect may be due to the effectiveness of the treatment – or possibly some other cause. In order to make this assessment, we need to calculate a **test statistic** and use this to determine the probability (expressed as a ***P*-value**). This process is called **hypothesis testing**.

At this point, it is useful to go back to the idea of the normal distribution and standard deviations. Remember that, in a normal distribution, 95% of all values fall within 1.96 standard deviations and 99% of them fall within 2.58 standard deviations.

If the value of a result is **more** than 1.96 standard deviations of the hypothetical or population mean value, its probability of occurring is less than 5%. Remembering (from Chapter 13) that probabilities are usually expressed as decimals, its probability is written as ***P* < 0.05** (< means 'less than'). If the value is more than 2.58 standard deviations away from the mean, its probability of occurring (if the H_0 is true) is less than 1%. Its probability is therefore ***P* < 0.01**. Probabilities of < 0.05 or < 0.01 are generally regarded as being the thresholds of **statistical significance**.

For many studies, a *P*-value of less than 0.05 is regarded as significant. For other more critical studies (e.g. treatment trials), significance may only be assigned when the *P*-value is < 0.01.

Our test statistic for comparing a sample mean with a hypothetical mean is calculated using the following relatively simple equation:

$$(\bar{x} - \mu)/\text{s.e.}$$

where $\bar{x}$ is the sample mean, μ is the **hypothetical** mean presumed in the H_0 and s.e. is the standard error of the observed value.

This test uses the normal distribution, and is thus called the **normal** test. It is also called the ***z*-test**.

Note: *the formula here should only be used for large samples – see Chapter 15 on t-tests if the sample size is small.*

The equation calculates the number of standard deviations that separate the hypothetical mean from the sample mean, and expresses this as something called a ***z*-score** (or **normal score**). The *z*-score is the test statistic that is used in the normal test. The larger the *z*-score, the smaller the probability of the null hypothesis being true.

The final step is to look up this *z*-score in a **normal distribution table** (either one-tailed or two-tailed, depending on the hypothesis) in order to obtain a *P*-value. An example of a normal distribution table for two-tailed hypotheses is provided in Appendix 1.

We know that 95% of all values under the normal distribution are contained within 1.96 standard deviations of the mean, and 99% of values are contained within 2.58 standard deviations. If the *z*-score is **more than 1.96**, we instantly know that the probability is less than 5%, and its *P*-value will therefore be < 0.05. If the *z*-score is **more than 2.58**, the probability is less than 1%, and its *P*-value will therefore be < 0.01.

The steps for the first equation on page 46 $(\bar{x} - \mu)$/s.e. are as follows:

1. Calculate the sample mean and standard error.
2. Subtract the hypothetical mean from the sample mean (ignore any minus values, since we are only interested in the **difference** between the two means).
3. Divide the result by the standard error to produce a *z*-score.
4. Look down each column of the normal distribution table in Appendix 1 to find your *z*-score, and then read across to obtain the *P*-value (e.g. for a *z*-score of 0.37, the *P*-value is 0.7114).

Many statistical computer programs produce *P*-values automatically, and it is possible that you will never actually need to calculate one.

Using the table of diastolic blood pressure readings in Chapter 12, we calculate a *P*-value as follows:

Suppose the **population** mean diastolic blood pressure in patients with diabetes is believed to be 84 mmHg.

1. The sample mean is 82.696 and the standard error is 1.116.
2. 82.696 – 84 = 1.304 (ignoring the minus value).
3. 1.304/1.116 = 1.17.
4. *z* = 1.17; in a two-tailed normal distribution table, look up 1.17 in the left-hand column, and then read across to find the *P*-value. The *P*-value = 0.2420, which is not significant. The null hypothesis (in this case, that there is no difference between the sample and the population) is **not** rejected. In fact, this sample could have come from a population with a mean blood pressure of 84 mmHg.

Now imagine that the diastolic blood pressures were taken from a group of men who have hypertension, and who have received a new antihypertensive drug in a certain clinic. We shall also assume that the population mean diastolic blood pressure in hypertensive men (whose blood pressure is either controlled or kept at a safe level by conventional drugs) aged 30–45 years who attend hypertension clinics is in fact 86 mmHg ((82.696 – 86)/1.116) = 3.304/1.116 = 2.96.

The *z*-score is now 2.96. The two-tailed normal distribution table gives a *P*-value of 0.0031. Thus the probability of this result being obtained if the null hypothesis (that there is no difference between the treatments) were true is very low. In this case, the null hypothesis will be rejected, and the alternative hypothesis (that there **is** a difference) will be accepted. It may be concluded that this drug is either highly effective, or that the result may have been influenced by another factor. Such factors could include problems with the sampling/randomisation process, differences between groups of patients receiving the treatments (either at the start of the study or with regard to patient management during the study) or the deliberate 'fiddling' of results.

It is worthwhile using a certain amount of common sense when interpreting P-values. A P-value of 0.6672 is certainly not significant, but a value of 0.0524 should not necessarily be dismissed just because it is slightly higher than the threshold. However, a P-value of 0.0524 will always be referred to and reported as non-significant.

A P-value of less than our chosen threshold of significance does not **prove** the null hypothesis to be true – it merely demonstrates insufficient evidence to reject it. There is always an element of uncertainty when using a P-value to decide whether or not to reject the null hypothesis.

When interpreting a P-value, two different types of possible error should be recognised:

- **type 1 error** – rejecting a **true** null hypothesis, and accepting a false alternative hypothesis
- **type 2 error** – **not** rejecting a **false** null hypothesis.

It is also worth remembering that a statistically significant result is not necessarily **clinically** significant. For example, a reduction in the mean diastolic blood pressure from 115 mmHg to 110 mmHg in a large sample of adults may well produce a P-value of < 0.05. However, a diastolic blood pressure of 110 mmHg is still well above what is considered to be a healthy level.

Although P-values are routinely calculated, there is a strength of feeling that confidence intervals may be a better way of testing hypotheses, since they show an estimate of where the true value actually lies. If a confidence interval does **not** include the hypothetical mean, this indicates significance. When reporting results, it is good practice to quote both P-values **and** confidence intervals.

There are different formulae for calculating z-scores in other situations (e.g. differences between proportions), and these are covered by several other texts.

CHAPTER 15

The *t*-tests

The previous methods of calculating confidence intervals and performing hypothesis testing are only suitable if the sample size is large. However, in some circumstances only small samples are available. For these purposes, a 'small' sample is usually considered to be 30 or less.

A different distribution – the ***t*-distribution** (also known as Student's *t*-distribution, after WS Gossett, whose pseudonym was 'Student') – is used if the sample size is small. The *t*-distribution has a similarly shaped curve to the normal distribution, but is more widely spread out and flatter. The degree of spread and flatness changes according to the sample size. If the sample size is very large, the *t*-distribution becomes virtually identical to the normal distribution. The *t*-tests are therefore suitable for both large and small sample sizes.

For the use of a *t*-test to be valid, the data should be normally distributed. Although the test is described as 'robust', meaning that it can withstand moderate departures from normality, severely skewed data are unsuitable. For independent tests, the standard deviations should also be roughly equal.

If you are in doubt as to whether the degree of skewedness of your data violates these conditions, statistical methods exist to assess this (*see* Chapter 16). There are also methods of transforming skewed data to make them more 'normal'. One alternative method for dealing with skew is to use a non-parametric test (*see* Chapter 17). For small samples, the Wilcoxon signed-rank test can be used instead of the paired *t*-test, and the Wilcoxon rank-sum test or Mann–Whitney *U*-test can be used instead of the independent *t*-test. These methods are covered by many more detailed texts.

The calculation of the *t*-statistic (*t*) is a little different to the calculation of *z*. It takes the level of significance (e.g. 0.05, 0.01) into account, together with **degrees of freedom (d.f.)** which are based on sample size. Don't worry too much about the theory behind degrees of freedom.

Degrees of freedom are calculated as follows:

$n - 1$ for a one-sample test

where n = sample size

$(n_1 - 1) + (n_2 - 1)$ for an independent test

where n_1 = sample size for group 1 and n_2 = sample size for group 2.

The steps for performing a t-test are as follows:

1. Work out the standard error and t-statistic for the required test.
2. Calculate the appropriate d.f.
3. Using the t-distribution table (*see* Appendix 1), look up the d.f. value in the left-hand column.
4. Read across this row, until the nearest values to the left and right of your t-statistic can be seen.
5. Your P-value will be **less than** the P-value at the top of the column to the left of your t-statistic and **greater than** the P-value at the top of the column to its right (e.g. a t-statistic of 2.687 with 6 d.f. falls in between 2.447 and 3.143. The nearest value to its left is 2.447; the P-value at the top of this column is 0.05. The P-value for your t-statistic will therefore be **less than** 0.05, and is written $P < 0.05$. If your t-statistic is 1.325 with 6 d.f., there is no column to its left, so the P-value will be **greater** than the column to its right, and is therefore > 0.2).

There are a number of different t-test formulae which are used in different situations, described as follows:

ONE-SAMPLE *T*-TEST

This test compares a sample mean with a population mean.

$t = (\bar{x} - \mu)/\text{s.e.}$

where $\bar{x}$ = sample mean, μ = population mean and s.e. = standard error of sample mean.

d.f. = $n - 1$

where n = sample size.

Calculating standard deviation and standard error for the independent *t*-test

If the standard deviations are not appreciably different, use the 'pooled' standard error:

$$\text{s.e. pooled} = \sqrt{\frac{s\text{ pooled}^2}{n_1} + \frac{s\text{ pooled}^2}{n_2}}$$

where s pooled is calculated in the formula following, n_1 = sample size 1 and n_2 = sample size 2.

To calculate a 'pooled' standard deviation:

$$s\text{ pooled} = \sqrt{\frac{[s_1^2(n_1-1)]+[s_2^2(n_2-1)]}{(n_1+n_2)-2}}$$

where s_1 = standard deviation 1, s_2 = standard deviation 2, n_1 = sample size 1 and n_2 = sample size 2.

If the standard deviations and/or sample sizes **are** appreciably different, it is advisable to consult a statistician or someone with advanced statistical skills.

95% Confidence intervals – independent *t*-test

$$\bar{x} + t_{0.05} \times \text{s.e. pooled}$$

where $t_{0.05}$ = value on *t*-distribution table in 0.05 column (two-tailed), corresponding to appropriate d.f.

$$\text{s.e.} = s/\sqrt{n}$$

where s = standard deviation of sample mean and n = sample size.

95% Confidence intervals – one-sample *t*-test

$$\bar{x} \pm t_{0.05} \times \text{s.e.}$$

where $t_{0.05}$ = value on *t*-distribution table in 0.05 column (two-tailed), corresponding to appropriate d.f.

For example, suppose that a group of 14 GP surgeries is running healthy eating groups to help patients to lose weight. At the start, each patient has their height measured and is weighed, and their body mass index (BMI) is calculated. The mean BMI is roughly the same for patients at each GP surgery. After 6 months, each patient is weighed and their BMI is recorded again. One surgery is interested to find out how successful its patients have been in losing weight, compared with the whole group. The BMI values of its patients are shown in Figure 15.1.

```
BMI value | Frequency
--------- + ---------
   21     |     1
   22     |     1
   26     |     1
   29     |     1
   30     |     2
   31     |     1
   32     |     1
   33     |     1
   35     |     1
--------- + ---------
  Total   |    10
```

Mean = 28.9
SD = 4.581

FIGURE 15.1 Frequency distribution of BMI from a sample of patients in primary care.

The mean BMI for the 14 surgeries as a whole is 26.2 (this is a precisely known population value), compared with 28.9 for this surgery. It looks as if this surgery's patients have been less successful, but has their performance been **significantly** different? Let us find out, by performing a one-sample *t*-test.

The steps are as follows:

1. Work out the standard error (n is 10; s is 4.581; $\sqrt{10}$ = 3.162): 4.581/3.162 = 1.449. The sample mean minus the population mean = 28.9 – 26.2 = 2.7. To work out the *t*-statistic: 2.7/1.449 = 1.863 (to three decimal places here).

2. Calculate the degrees of freedom (d.f.): $10 - 1 = 9$.

3–5. Using the t-distribution table, look up d.f. = 9, and then read across this row. Our t-statistic is in between 1.833 and 2.262. Reading up the columns for these two values shows that the corresponding two-tailed P-value is less than 0.1 but greater than 0.05, and is therefore not significant.

The null hypothesis (in this case, that there is no difference between the BMI values in this GP surgery and the group as a whole) is **not** rejected.

To calculate a 95% confidence interval, the steps are as follows:

1. Note the sample mean, standard error and degrees of freedom.
2. Find the value in the two-tailed t-distribution table in the 0.05 column, corresponding to the degrees of freedom.
3. Multiply this value by the standard error, and note the result (call it **result 1**).
4. Add **result 1** to the mean, and note this sum (call it *sum a*).
5. Subtract **result 1** from the mean, and note this sum (call it *sum b*).
6. The confidence interval is written as:

   95% c.i. = (sample mean) ((*sum a*) → (*sum b*)).

Using the mentioned example, the steps are as follows:

1. The sample mean is 28.9, the standard error is 1.449 and there are 9 degrees of freedom.
2. In the t-distribution table in Appendix 1, find degrees of freedom = 9, and then read along the line until you come to the 0.05 column – the value is 2.262.
3. Multiply 2.262 by the standard error ($2.262 \times 1.449 = 3.278$) (**result 1**).
4. $28.9 + 3.278 = 32.178$ (*sum a*).
5. $28.9 - 3.278 = 25.622$ (*sum b*).
6. 95% c.i. = 28.9 (25.622 → 32.178).

Note that the confidence interval includes the mean of the group as a whole (26.2). This supports the null hypothesis that there is no difference between the BMI values.

PAIRED (ALSO CALLED THE DEPENDENT) *T*-TEST

This test is used to assess the difference between two **paired** measurements. It tests the null hypothesis that the mean of the difference is zero. In this case, data are naturally paired or matched (e.g. weight measurements from the **same subjects** at a 6-month interval or data relative to twins or couples).

The value that we analyse for each pair is the *difference* between the two measurements.

$$t = \bar{x}/\text{s.e.}$$

where $\bar{x}$ = mean of the differences and s.e. = standard error of the differences.

$$\text{d.f.} = n - 1$$

where n = sample size.

$$\text{s.e.} = s/\sqrt{n}$$

where s = standard deviation of the differences and n = sample size.

95% Confidence intervals – paired *t*-test

$$\bar{x} \pm t_{0.05} \times \text{s.e.}$$

where $t_{0.05}$ = value on t-distribution table in 0.05 column (two-tailed), correspond to appropriate d.f.

INDEPENDENT (ALSO CALLED THE TWO-SAMPLE OR UNPAIRED) *T*-TES

This is used where data are collected from groups which are unrelated (or indep ent), such as the length at 1 year of a group of infants who were breastfed, comp with a group who were not breastfed.

$$t = (\bar{x}_1 - \bar{x}_2)/\text{s.e. pooled}$$

where $\bar{x}_1$ = mean from group 1 and $\bar{x}_2$ = mean from group 2.

$$\text{d.f.} = (n_1 - 1) + (n_2 - 1)$$

where n_1 = sample size for group 1 and n_2 = sample size for group 2.

s.e. pooled = see following.

CHAPTER 16

Data checking

Once your data have been collected, it is natural to want to get on with the job of analysis. Before going any further however, it is absolutely essential to check the data thoroughly. The process of data checking can be tiresome, but ignoring it may lead to your drawing the wrong conclusions. This chapter provides a brief overview of some of the issues to be considered.

PREVENTION IS BETTER THAN CURE

The best advice is to think carefully about your data before you get anywhere near the analysis stage – both in the planning of a study and during data collection. Piloting your data collection instrument before the study begins can help to minimise 'bugs' and possible misunderstandings by both participants and researchers. Thinking in advance about potential biases and problems can help to reduce data errors – this can save considerable time and distress later on (*see also* Chapter 28 on Questionnaires). Data entry can be tedious and requires concentration and alertness, so taking care to enter data accurately can also pay dividends. You could check a sample of data as you go along, or even ask someone else to check some or all of what has been entered before doing your analysis (discussed further below).

When reviewing data, it is helpful to ask yourself the following questions:

HAVE THE DATA BEEN ENTERED ACCURATELY?

This includes checking that the data have been accurately recorded and entered. It is helpful to 'eyeball' the data to check that the data set looks right. Typing errors are common and easily made, so it is good practice to check that data have been entered correctly by comparing the records used for data entry with what appears in your database. Some software packages allow automated checking of data validity. Of course, any changes to your data should only be made where an actual mistake has been identified.

ARE THERE ANY MISSING DATA?

In the real world, it is difficult to achieve 100% completeness. For example, some participants may refuse to answer certain questions or fail to complete all fields in a questionnaire, others may leave a study for various reasons or some practices may not keep records of every variable you want to collect data for.

Where data are incomplete, you need to decide how best to act. It is possible (though unlikely) that you could attempt to go back to collect the missing data; this will be impossible if your subjects were anonymous, but may be feasible under some circumstances and if time allows. If the missing data have arisen from errors in data entry, this should be straightforward to correct as described previously. However, if this cannot be done, you could continue with one of the following options:

- Analyse what you have anyway. This may be acceptable if relatively small amounts of data are missing, but large quantities of missing data could seriously undermine the reliability of your results. Be aware that sample size would be affected. You would need to report the fact that data were missing, and discuss how this may affect your results
- Exclude the incomplete variable(s) from your analysis. If the variables concerned are not very important to your analysis and not central to answering a research question, this may be a viable option. Otherwise, the missing data may present a major problem that could ruin your whole study. If this is the case, you could consider estimating missing values – see the next point
- Estimate the missing values. This may be possible using various techniques such as dummy variables or applying mean values or other methods that estimate or impute missing values. These should always be used with care, preferably with the help of a statistician, and are not covered by this basic guide. When estimated values have been substituted for missing data, it is a good idea to carry out separate analyses on the variable both with missing data **and** with substituted data – in this case, both results should be reported, with discussion on the differences between results, where this is relevant.

If you draft a report using incomplete data and add further entries later, it is important to check the draft against your **final** analysis – you otherwise risk inconsistencies and errors in your report (Smeeton & Goda, 2003).

ARE THERE ANY OUTLIERS?

These are values that are either extremely high or extremely low. We have already seen in Chapters 7 and 9 that such extreme values can lead to misleading results, so your data set should be carefully checked for outliers. These may arise from errors in data provided by study participants or from data entry mistakes – or an extreme value could be real. Sometimes, an outlier can affect more than one variable. For example, if an extreme weight value was recorded, and weight will be used to calculate a separate BMI variable.

To check for outliers, you can either look at the range of a variable (the lowest and highest values) or produce a graph showing all the values, such as a histogram, for checking the range, or scatterplots for looking at the relationship between two values, e.g. weight and height, to see if they appear to be consistent with each other.

Some outliers are obviously erroneous (e.g. a human age of 240 years is definitely wrong), while others could actually be genuine (e.g. a male weight of 240 kg is very heavy, but possible). In either case, it is advisable to go back to the original data and check whether the outlier appears real. If you are sure that an error has been made and can identify the correct value, you can amend it. Careful judgement must be used when doing this, however, as it would clearly be inappropriate and unethical to delete or change a value just because it seemed wrong.

If you are unsure about whether to delete an outlier, you could (as with missing data, discussed earlier) carry out two analyses – one with the outlier left in and another with it deleted, to see how large an effect this has on your results. If the results are very different, you should consider employing more advanced statistical methods such as transformation and non-parametric tests to deal with this (Petrie & Sabin, 2009). In the latter case, it is advisable to seek expert statistical advice.

ARE THE DATA NORMALLY DISTRIBUTED?

Statistical tests make 'assumptions' (or have requirements) about the kind of data they can be used with, and often require that the data are normally distributed. For example, we have seen an assumption for using t-tests is that the data are normally distributed.

If data **are** normally distributed, we can use **parametric** statistical tests (such as a t-test) to analyse the data (note – there may still be unsatisfied assumptions that invalidate them, e.g. unequal variances in an independent samples t-test). For data that are **not** normally distributed, there are various broadly comparable techniques called **non-parametric** tests – for example, the Wilcoxon signed-rank test is a non-parametric equivalent of the paired t-test. There is some more detail on this in the next chapter.

The problem is that non-parametric tests are less likely to show statistical significance when there is a real difference – the risk of a type 2 error is usually greater with a non-parametric test, so technically they tend to be less powerful. Also, parametric tests and their non-parametric equivalents do not always test the same hypothesis (e.g. paired *t*-tests test for equal means, while Wilcoxon signed-rank tests for equal medians). It is therefore always better to use parametric tests if possible.

As part of the process of screening data before carrying out analysis, we can use tests such as the Kolmogorov–Smirnov or the Shapiro–Wilk to find out whether the data are normally distributed.

When we have data that are not normally distributed, we can try transforming the data – this is done in an attempt to 'normalise' them (i.e. transform them into normally distributed data), so that we can use a parametric test. A commonly used transformation is the logarithmic/$\log_{10}$, though there is a range of others that can be used. Transformation may or may not succeed in normalising the data. If we transform a variable, and it is then identified as 'normally distributed', we can more safely use a parametric test to analyse it. If the transformation does not normalise the data, we should use an appropriate non-parametric test instead.

Although you can visually inspect the data, for example, by using a histogram (Petrie & Sabin, 2009), to check whether it resembles the symmetrical bell-shaped pattern described in Chapter 11, normality is often checked using one of two just previously mentioned tests:

- **Kolmogorov–Smirnov** – for large samples (e.g. 50 or more)
- **Shapiro–Wilk** – best for sample sizes of **less than** 50.

When using these tests, the **null hypothesis** is that the distribution **is** normally distributed.

This means that:

- if $P < 0.05$, we reject the null hypothesis and conclude that the data are **not** normally distributed
- if $P \geq 0.05$, the data are not significantly non-normal, so may be assumed normally distributed.

The Q–Q plot (abbreviation of 'quantile–quantile' plot, produced by some programs) can also be used to check normality. If the data are normally distributed, the dots should fall along the straight line on the plot.

If our statistical testing will involve comparing groups, then the data for each group should be checked for normality. Some care needs to be taken when using these tests of normality, as they can be unreliable under certain circumstances. It is therefore advisable to also use Q–Q plots when interpreting them (Field, 2013).

Transformation and normality tests are performed using computer programs, and instructions for carrying them out differ between various packages.

Let's now look at two examples of normality tests with abbreviated outputs produced by SPSS Statistics software.

First, we are going to check the normality of systolic blood pressure readings from a group of patients, which have been entered onto a database. The following output is produced:

Tests of normality

	Kolmogorov–Smirnov			Shapiro–Wilk		
	Statistic	df	Sig.	Statistic	df	Sig.
Systolic blood pressure (mmHg)	.123	39	.002	.967	39	.021

A total of 39 systolic readings are recorded (a 'small' sample size), so we will use the Shapiro–Wilk test.

We can see that the *P*-value (shown as 'Sig.' in the table) is **0.021** – this is < 0.05, so indicates that systolic blood pressure is **not** normally distributed.

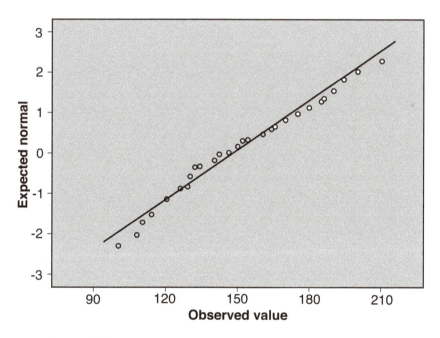

FIGURE 16.1 Normal Q–Q plot of systolic blood pressure (mmHg).

Looking at the Q–Q plot shown in Figure 16.1, we can see that the dots are **not** arranged along the straight line, which confirms that systolic blood pressure is not normally distributed. Although they may seem to be quite close to the line, the data swing a few points under the line (the lowest observed values), then several over, then do another run under. For normality, the points should be close to the line.

For the second example, we will use the database of Warwick-Edinburgh Mental Well-being Scale (WEMWBS) scores for mental well-being used in Chapter 22 on effect size. A total of 60 scores are recorded for patients receiving the 'new therapy' and the output looks like this:

Tests of normality

	Kolmogorov–Smirnov			Shapiro–Wilk		
	Statistic	df	Sig.	Statistic	df	Sig.
New Therapy WEMWBS	.085	60	.200	.982	60	.526

A total of 60 WEMWBS scores are recorded (a 'large' sample size), so this time we will use the Kolmogorov–Smirnov test.

This time, we can see that the P-value is **0.200** – this is > 0.05, so there is no reason to reject the assumption that these scores are normally distributed.

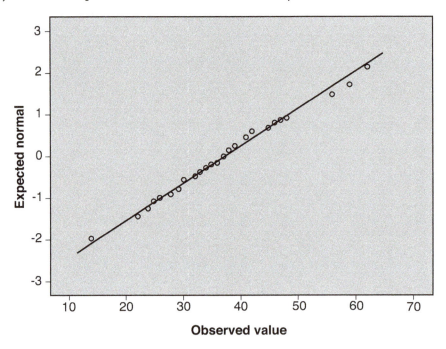

FIGURE 16.2 Normal Q–Q plot of baseline.

Looking at the Q-Q plot shown in Figure 16.2, we can see that the dots are generally arranged along the straight line (much more closely than in the previous example), which suggests that these baseline WEMWBS scores are normally distributed.

THE CENTRAL LIMIT THEOREM

So far in this chapter, we have discussed the importance of checking your data for normality using formal methods (such as the Kolmogorov–Smirnov or Shapiro–Wilk tests and Q–Q plots) as a prerequisite for using parametric statistical techniques.

Having read this, it may surprise you to know that something called the **central limit theorem** says that as long as your sample size is reasonably large (say 20 or more), you can probably proceed as if the distribution is normal.

The central limit theorem was first proposed over 200 years ago, and is about what happens to the sample mean 'in the limit' when the sample size heads off towards infinity. It has since been shown that it is practically true for means of fairly small samples (in practice, sometimes even < 10) if the shape of the distribution for the **individual measurements** is not normal but is in some sense 'reasonable'. In practice therefore, even if a test of normality such as Shapiro–Wilk shows that the data for a sample of say 20 or 30 are significantly non-normal, the sampling distribution of the mean will be very close to normal, and hence most standard parametric tests will be valid, unless the distribution is very skewed. This will, however, not be true of tests that do not relate to the mean.

This does not suggest that you should ignore parametric assumptions and testing for normality, but the central limit theorem should be borne in mind if, for example, you only have a small data set and wish to use a parametric analysis technique.

CHAPTER 17

Parametric and non-parametric tests

People often ask about the difference between parametric and non-parametric tests. We introduced the concept of **parameters** early in the book – these are measures of a population, rather than of a sample. Used in this context, the term refers to the 'population' of the normal distribution. Parametric tests are performed if a normal distribution can be assumed. Remember that the t-tests also require an underlying normal distribution.

However, if the data are clearly not normally distributed, **non-parametric tests** can be used. These are also known as **distribution-free tests**, and they include the following:

- Wilcoxon signed-rank test – **replaces the paired t-test**
- Mann–Whitney U-test **or** Wilcoxon rank-sum test – **replaces the independent t-test**
- Chi-squared (χ^2) test – **for categorical data**
- Spearman's (Spearman's ρ or rho) rank correlation coefficient – **replaces Pearson's product moment correlation coefficient**
- Kendall's τ (or tau) – **alternative to Spearman's rho** (bullet point 4)
- Kruskal–Wallis test – **replaces one-way analysis of variance (ANOVA)**.

The Chi-squared test is described in Chapter 20. The other tests are covered by several other statistical textbooks (*see* Further reading).

CHAPTER 18

Correlation and linear regression

Various statistical methods exist for investigating association between variables. In the next two chapters, we will be looking at the Chi-squared (χ^2) test (used for investigating the presence of an association between categorical variables), as well as briefly outlining multiple regression, logistic regression, and analysis of variance (ANOVA). This chapter, however, concentrates on methods for assessing possible association, mainly between **continuous** variables.

CORRELATION

Correlation assesses the **strength** of association between variables (usually interval or ratio), and **linear regression** allows us to use one variable to predict another.

Let's have a look at how we can put this into practice. A rheumatologist measures and records the bone mineral density (BMD) in a group of women. She has a hypothesis that BMD decreases with age, and decides to use correlation and linear regression to explore this.

Correlation is measured using a **correlation coefficient** (*r*), which can take any value between −1 and +1. If $r = +1$, there is a **perfect positive correlation**; if $r = −1$ there is a **perfect negative correlation**; a value of $r = 0$ represents **no linear correlation** (we will discuss what is meant by **linear** in a moment). It follows that if *r* is more than 0 but less than +1, there is **imperfect positive correlation**, and if *r* is more than −1 but less than 0, there is **imperfect negative correlation**. If we plot the age and BMD data on a scatterplot (*see* page 11 for more information on scatterplots), the shape that the dots form will give us a clue about the relationship between age and BMD. If, for example, there is a **perfect positive correlation**, BMD **increases** with age ($r = +1$), and the scatterplot will appear as shown in Figure 18.1.

Each dot on the graph represents an individual's age (shown on the *x*-axis) and their BMD value (on the *y*-axis). Note that age is the independent variable (since our hypothesis is that BMD depends on age, age is independent of any influence from

BMD), and is thus placed on the *x*-axis. This makes BMD the dependent variable, which is placed on the *y*-axis. You can see that the dots form a straight line, showing a **linear relationship** between the two variables.

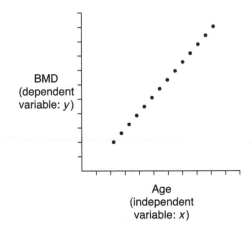

FIGURE 18.1 Scatterplot showing a perfect positive correlation between age and BMD.

If, on the other hand, there is **perfect negative correlation**, BMD decreases with age, $r = -1$, and the scatterplot will look as it does in Figure 18.2.

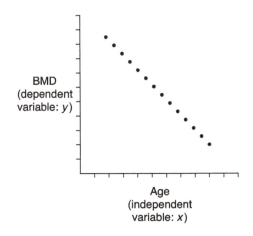

FIGURE 18.2 Scatterplot showing a perfect negative correlation between age and BMD.

If there is no linear correlation at all between age and BMD ($r = 0$), the scatterplot may resemble that in Figure 18.3. In this figure, you can see that there is no discernible linear relationship between age and BMD.

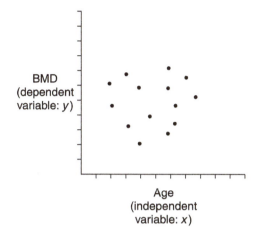

FIGURE 18.3 Scatterplot showing no linear correlation between age and BMD.

There might be an **imperfect correlation** (either positive or negative). Figure 18.4 shows an **imperfect positive correlation**, where BMD increases with age, but where r is somewhere between 0 and +1 (quite close to +1, in fact). A fairly strong and clear linear relationship can be seen, but the dots do not lie in a straight line, as in perfect correlation.

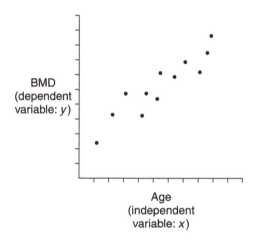

FIGURE 18.4 Scatterplot showing an imperfect positive correlation between age and BMD.

There could also be an imperfect negative correlation, as can be seen in Figure 18.5. In this case, r would be quite close to –1.

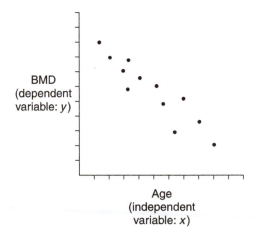

FIGURE 18.5 Scatterplot showing an imperfect negative correlation between age and BMD.

Finally, there may be a **non-linear relationship**, one example of which is shown in Figure 18.6.

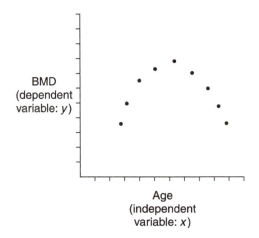

FIGURE 18.6 Scatterplot showing a non-linear relationship between age and BMD.

Correlation is often calculated using the Pearson's product moment correlation coefficient (commonly known as **Pearson's ρ**), the formula for which is:

$$r = \frac{\Sigma(x-\bar{x})(y-\bar{y})}{\sqrt{\Sigma(x-\bar{x})^2 \, \Sigma(y-\bar{y})^2}}$$

where: x = individual exposure $\bar{x}$ = mean exposure
        y = individual outcome $\bar{y}$ = mean outcome

Do not worry if this equation looks complicated! All of the calculations can easily be done by computer, so you should never need to work this out by hand. It is important, however, that you understand some of the theory behind this process, and know how to interpret the computer outputs that are generated.

This formula should only be used when:

- there is no clear **non-linear** relationship between the variables
- only one value is recorded for each patient (e.g. observations are independent, **not** paired – *see* paired *t*-test in Chapter 15).

Coming back to our example, let's use Pearson's product moment correlation coefficient to find the strength of association between age and BMD. The data collected by our consultant rheumatologist are shown in Table 18.1.

TABLE 18.1 Age and BMD data for 10 patients

Age	BMD
46	1.112
49	0.916
52	0.989
56	0.823
58	0.715
60	0.817
64	0.834
68	0.726
75	0.654
79	0.612

In real life we would hope to use a much larger sample than 10 patients, but we will just regard this as an example to illustrate the techniques we are studying. First of all, let us plot the data (Figure 18.7).

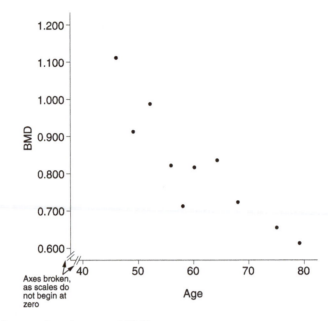

FIGURE 18.7 Scatterplot of age and BMD.

Note that each axis in the figure has been broken using two parallel lines, to denote that the scale does not begin at 0. The shape of the dots on the scatterplot shows an imperfect negative correlation between age and BMD (compare this with Figure 18.5). BMD does indeed appear to generally decrease with age. This alone, however, is not enough to demonstrate a correlation and test significance – for this we need to calculate Pearson's product moment correlation coefficient.

When the data are analysed using a computer program (in this case, SPSS Statistics version 22.0 (IBM Corporation, 2013)), the following output is produced (other computer programs may produce different looking outputs, but the results are equivalent):

Correlations

		Age	BMD
Age	Pearson correlation	1	−.891**
	Sig. (2-tailed)		.001
	N	10	10
BMD	Pearson correlation	−.891**	1
	Sig. (2-tailed) correlation	.001	
	N	10	10

**Correlation is significant at the 0.01 level

Although the output does not specifically include the symbol 'r', it shows that the Pearson correlation (coefficient) is –0.891, and that the two-tailed significance (P-value) is 0.001. Don't worry about the fact that both of these figures seem to be shown twice (one for age and BMD, the other for BMD and age) on the output. The correlation coefficient (r) is –0.891, which is more than –1, but less than 0. The figure of –0.891 is quite close to the maximum value of –1, and therefore indicates a relatively strong correlation between age and BMD.

When assessing the strength of an association using r, 0 to 0.19 is regarded as very weak, 0.2 to 0.39 weak, 0.40 to 0.59 moderate, 0.6 to 0.79 strong and 0.8 to 1 very strong (Swinscow & Campbell, 2002). These values can be plus or minus. These labels are useful, though somewhat arbitrary. Our value of –0.891 would therefore be regarded as 'very strong'.

The figure 'Sig.' represents the P-value of 0.001, indicating a significant correlation. We can therefore conclude that there is a **significant** negative correlation between age and BMD in women, and can accept the consultant rheumatologist's hypothesis that BMD decreases as age increases.

We can also calculate r^2 – this indicates how much variation in one variable can be explained by the other. If we square r, we get –0.891 × –0.891 = 0.794. This means that age is responsible for 0.794 (or 79.4%) of the total variation in BMD. This does **not** mean, however, that age **causes** the variation in BMD (the subject of causality is discussed in Chapter 26).

If Pearson's product moment correlation coefficient cannot be used (e.g. if there is no clear linear relationship – see previously listed criteria), it might be appropriate to employ **Spearman's rank correlation coefficient**. This is the **non-parametric** version of Pearson's product moment correlation coefficient, and is also called **Spearman's ρ** or **Spearman's rho**. It can be used when any of the following apply:

- there is a small sample size
- there is no clear **linear** relationship between the variables
- one or both variables are ordinal.

We have a small sample size in our age and BMD study, so in this case it is also appropriate to use the Spearman's rank correlation coefficient. When calculated, the following SPSS output is produced:

Correlations

			Age	BMD
Spearman's rho	Age	Correlation coefficient	1.000	−.867**
		Sig. (2-tailed)	.	.001
		N	10	10
	BMD	Correlation coefficient	−.867**	1.000
		Sig. (2-tailed)	.001	.
		N	10	10

**Correlation is significant at the 0.01 level (2-tailed)

This shows that although the correlation coefficient is slightly smaller than when using Pearson's product moment correlation coefficient (−0.867 compared to −0.891), the result is still significant.

Kendall's τ (also called **Kendall's tau**) can be used as an alternative to Spearman's rank correlation coefficient. This is covered in other texts – *see* Further reading.

So we have demonstrated the presence of a strong (and statistically significant) correlation between age and BMD in women.

LINEAR REGRESSION

As mentioned at the start of the chapter, we can also use **linear regression** to predict the value of BMD for any specific age. This is achieved by calculating a straight line that best fits the association. This line is called the **linear regression line**. The line describes how much the value of one variable changes when the other variable increases or decreases.

Linear regression should only be used when all of the following assumptions apply:

- the observations are independent
- an imperfect linear relationship exists between x and y
- the value of y is normally distributed, for any value of x
- the size of the scatter of the points around the line is the same throughout the length of the line.

(In practice, the last two assumptions are difficult to determine; a statistician should be consulted if there is any doubt.)

The formula for the regression line is:

$$y = a + bx$$

These letters represent the following:

y = the variable on the y-axis
x = the variable on the x-axis
a = the intercept or constant (the value of y when $x = 0$)
b = the gradient of the line (the amount that y increases when x is increased by one
　　unit).

In fact, a and b are also known as the **regression coefficients**, and b is sometimes labelled B or β.

Going back to our example, we already know that y = BMD and x = AGE. So the equation $y = a + bx$ effectively says that: BMD = $a + (b \times AGE)$

All we need to know now are the regression coefficients, a and b.

We will use a computer program for our calculations. When a linear regression is performed using SPSS, a fairly lengthy output is produced, including the following table:

This is **a**

Model		Unstandardized coefficients		Standardized coefficients	t	Sig.
		B	Std. error	Beta		
1	(Constant)	1.588	.140		11.331	.000
	Age	−.013	.002	−.891	−5.559	.001

This is **b**

The coefficients have not actually been labelled as 'a' and 'b' in the table, so arrows indicating the regression coefficients, a and b have been added for clarity. There is no need for us to deal with the items of information that have been covered over in grey, though other textbooks discuss these in detail. We shall concentrate on the column labelled 'B'. As mentioned earlier, a is also known as the 'constant', which is shown in the table as 1.588. The other coefficient, b (labelled 'Age'), has a value of −0.013.

Our equation can now be completed:

$y = a + bx$
i.e. BMD = $a + (b \times AGE)$
i.e. BMD = $1.588 + (−0.013 \times AGE)$
i.e. BMD = $1.588 − (0.013 \times AGE)$

Imagine that we would like to **predict** the expected BMD for a woman aged 50. This could be calculated by inserting '50' for the age value:

BMD = 1.588 + (–0.013 × 50)
i.e. BMD = 1.588 + –0.65
i.e. BMD = 1.588 – 0.65
BMD = **0.938**

So an average woman aged 50 would have a predicted BMD of **0.938**. We can easily do the same for a woman aged 60:

BMD = 1.588 + (–0.013 × 60)
i.e. BMD = 1.588 + –0.78
i.e. BMD = 1.588 – 0.78
BMD = **0.808**

An average woman aged 60 would therefore have a predicted BMD of **0.808**.
And again for a woman aged 70:

BMD = 1.588 + (–0.013 × 70)
i.e. BMD = 1.588 + –0.91
i.e. BMD = 1.588 – 0.91
BMD = **0.678**

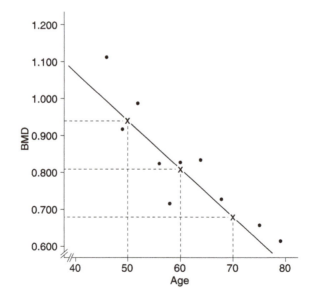

FIGURE 18.8 Scatterplot for age and BMD data, showing regression line.

An average woman aged 70 would therefore have a predicted BMD of **0.678**. The predicted BMD values for these ages are summarised in Table 18.2.

TABLE 18.2 Predicted BMD values for ages 50, 60 and 70

Age	Predicted BMD
50	0.938
60	0.808
70	0.678

Going back to our scatterplot, we can plot the three predicted BMD values, and join them up to show the regression line (Figure 18.8).

You may have noticed that the line does not actually go through any of the observed points.

For each of the three predicted values, dotted lines have been drawn upwards from age, then across from BMD value. An 'x' is marked where each intersects. A line has then been drawn through the three xs, to form the **regression line**.

Linear regression is therefore a useful technique, which allows us to use one value to predict another.

CHAPTER 19

Analysis of variance and some other types of regression

When looking at z- and t-tests in earlier chapters, we were limited to comparing only one mean value with another. However, it is often useful to examine differences between more than two means. For example, we may want to examine whether the weight of infants at 1 year of age is influenced by any of six types of milk they have received since birth. The object of the study is to find out which type of milk will produce the greatest weight gain. If each type of milk is called formula 1, 2, 3, 4 and 5, and breast milk, a total of 15 comparisons of mean weight are possible:

TABLE 19.1 Possible combinations for five different types of formula milk compared with breast milk

Formula 1; formula 2	Formula 2; formula 3	Formula 3; formula 5	Formula 1; formula 5	Formula 1; breast milk
Formula 1; formula 3	Formula 2; formula 4	Formula 3; breast milk	Formula 2; breast milk	Formula 3; formula 4
Formula 1; formula 4	Formula 2; formula 5	Formula 4; formula 5	Formula 4; breast milk	Formula 5; breast milk

Performing a separate z- or t-test for every possible combination would therefore require 15 separate tests. Besides being very time-consuming, such repeated testing is likely to produce statistically significant results which are misleading. A P-value of 0.05 or less would be expected from 5% (1 in 20) of all tests performed when there are no real differences (Kirkwood, 1988). This probability is increased if repeated tests are performed. With 15 tests, the chance of getting at least one wrong conclusion is therefore more than 50%. In other words, we have a greater risk of making a type 1 error – rejecting at least one true null hypothesis, and accepting a false alternative hypothesis.

A technique called **analysis of variance** or **ANOVA** allows several groups to be compared in one **single** statistical test, and indicates whether any significant differences exist between them.

The mentioned example compares mean weight at 1 year of age with the six groups (type of milk used). In other words, the numerical outcome variable (weight) is being compared to **one** categorical exposure group (type of milk). In this situation, **one-way** ANOVA can be used.

Where **two or more** categorical exposure groups need to be included (e.g. type of milk and ethnic group), then **two-way** ANOVA needs to be used. Details of two-way and other types of ANOVA are not covered by this basic guide, but are discussed in other texts – *see* Further reading. This chapter will therefore concentrate on **one-way ANOVA**.

The calculation of one-way ANOVA is normally carried out using a computer program. It assumes that data in each group are normally distributed, with equal standard deviations. This can be checked using techniques such as **Levene's test** (it can often be carried out by programs at the same time as one-way ANOVA). If the assumptions are not met, the **non-parametric** version of one-way ANOVA – the **Kruskal–Wallis test** – should be used instead.

One-way ANOVA compares the variance (this is the square of the standard deviation – *see* Chapter 9) of the means **between the groups** with the variance of the subjects **within the groups**, and uses the F-test to check for differences between these two variances. The null hypothesis is that variances between the groups are due to chance, and hence the outcome is **not** influenced by differences between the exposure categories. A P-value of < 0.05 would suggest that the outcome **is** influenced by differences between the exposure categories.

In the example, a P-value of < 0.05 would indicate that weight at 1 year of age **was** significantly influenced by the type of milk used. Unfortunately, ANOVA does not tell us **which** type of milk produced the greatest weight gain – we would need to go back to the data and check the mean weight achieved for each group.

Let's try using one-way ANOVA with the help of a computer program. We have an electronic database containing the BMI (body mass index – a measurement of obesity) values of 433 patients living in a town which is made up of five localities – A, B, C, D and E – with differing levels of social deprivation. We are interested in finding out whether BMI levels are influenced by which locality people live in. In other words, whether people living in the most deprived localities are more likely to be obese.

The computer program is likely to require you to define which variable is **dependent** and which is **fixed**. In this case, we are hypothesising that people's BMI may be influenced by (or depend on) the locality in which they reside, so BMI is the **dependent variable**, and locality is 'fixed' – this is called the **factor**.

When a one-way ANOVA is performed using SPSS, an output is produced including the tables following. These have been edited for simplicity. There is no need for us to deal with any items of information that have been covered in grey, though other textbooks discuss these in detail.

| | | BMI value | |
		Mean	Count
Locality	A	26.1	71
	B	26.9	88
	C	29.6	68
	D	29.8	115
	E	30.5	91
	Total		433

This output table shows mean BMI values for each locality, along with a count (frequency) for each. It appears that people in the **least** deprived locality (A) have the lowest mean BMI value, while those having the highest BMI values reside in the **most** deprived locality (E). What we do not yet know, of course, is whether this effect is significant.

As mentioned previously, Levene's test can be used to test the assumptions of one-way ANOVA.

Levene's test of equality of error variances

F	df1	df2	Sig.
.409	4	428	.802
Tests the null hypothesis that the error variance of the dependent variable is equal across groups.			

In the output shown, we can ignore the information in the grey cells, and concentrate on the significance ('Sig.') column. This shows a non-significant P-value (**0.802**). There is no evidence that variances across the groups (and hence standard deviations) are unequal – it is therefore appropriate to use one-way ANOVA. If this P-value were significant (< 0.05), the Kruskal–Wallis test should be used instead.

The following is an example computer output for a one-way ANOVA.

Tests of between-subjects effects

Source	Type III sum of squares	df	Mean square	F	Sig.
Corrected model	1253.230	4	313.308	12.291	.000
Intercept	341257.428	1	341257.428	13387.065	.000
Locality	1253.230	4	313.308	12.291	.000
Error	10910.396	428	25.492		
Total	369275.000	433			
Corrected total	12163.626	432			

We only need to focus on the F-statistic (F) and significance (Sig.) for **locality**. The F-statistic is 12.291, and there is a significant P-value of 0.000, or < 0.0001. This P-value suggests that (in this town), BMI **is** influenced by which locality people reside in.

There are considerable similarities between ANOVA and multiple regression (mentioned briefly following), and the two techniques generally give equivalent results (Kirkwood & Sterne, 2003).

OTHER TYPES OF REGRESSION
Multiple regression

In the linear regression example earlier, we used only one 'exposure' variable: age. It is also possible to examine the effect of **more than** one exposure, using **multiple regression**. For example, we could look at the effects of three continuous variables: age, BMD **and** height.

It is possible that height is a factor that could influence the value of BMD, as well as age. We could call this a **confounding** factor (discussed further in Chapter 24). Multiple regression could tell us whether age and BMD are still related, even when height is taken into account. If this is so, we can assume that height is not acting as a confounding factor.

The assumptions for multiple regression are the same as for linear regression. Three or more continuous variables can be used, and it is also possible to include categorical variables (e.g. ethnic group or sex). It is best, however, to keep the number of variables fairly small.

This technique goes beyond 'basic' statistical methods, and is covered in other texts – *see* Further reading.

Logistic regression

This is a technique that uses dichotomous variables (e.g. yes/no, present/absent, male/female) to predict the probability of an outcome.

For example, a total of 303 alcohol-abusing men were studied, to ascertain whether diagnosis of liver cirrhosis could be made on the basis of clinical symptoms alone, without the need to perform a surgical liver biopsy (Hamberg *et al.*, 1996). Six symptoms were studied: facial telangiectasia, vascular spiders, white nails, abdominal wall veins, fatness and peripheral oedema. In this case, the 'dichotomous variables' were the symptoms (because patients either **have** or **do not have** a particular symptom) and the dichotomous 'outcome' was liver cirrhosis. **Logistic regression** was used to predict the likelihood that a person having any **combination** of the symptoms actually had liver cirrhosis. A concise explanation of the logistic regression analysis used in this study was subsequently published in *Bandolier* (Freeman, 1997), and is available online at: www.medicine.ox.ac.uk/bandolier/band37/b37-5.html Results of the analysis were used to predict that people who experienced **all six** symptoms had a 97% chance of having cirrhosis, whereas there was a 20% chance in those who only had white nails and fatness.

Further details on logistic regression can be found in other texts – *see* Further reading.

CHAPTER 20

Chi-squared test

So far we have looked at hypothesis tests for continuous variables, from which summary statistics such as means and medians can be calculated. However, when we have only categorical data, means and medians cannot be obtained. For example, it is not possible to calculate the mean of a group of colours.

The Chi-squared test (Chi is pronounced 'ki', as in 'kind' and is normally written as χ^2) overcomes this problem, allowing hypothesis testing for categorical data. For example, we may wish to determine whether passive smokers are more likely to develop circulatory disease than those who are not exposed to smoke. In this example, passive smoking is the exposure and circulatory disease is the outcome. The Chi-squared test is a non-parametric test (*see* Chapter 17).

A good way to start examining the data is to present them in an *r* × *c* **table** (row × column; also known as a **cross-classification** or **contingency table**). Data are presented in cells, arranged in rows (horizontal) and columns (vertical). These often appear in the form of a **2 × 2 table** (so called because it shows two exposures and two outcomes). An example of a 2 × 2 table is shown in Table 20.1.

TABLE 20.1 Example of a 2 × 2 table

		Outcome present?		
		Yes	No	Total
Exposure taken place?	Yes	*a*	*b*	*a* + *b*
	No	*c*	*d*	*c* + *d*
	Total	*a* + *c*	*b* + *d*	*a* + *b* + *c* + *d*

If there are more than two categories of either exposure or outcome, then the number of columns or rows is increased, and the table is called a **2 × n table**. More categories can be used if required, in an *r* × *c* (row × column) table. The test statistic is calculated by taking the frequencies that are actually **observed** (*O*) and then working out the frequencies which would be **expected** (**E**) if the null hypothesis was true. The hypothesis (H_1) will be that there is an association between the variables, and the null hypothesis (H_0) will be that there is no association between the variables.

The expected frequencies are calculated as follows:

$$\frac{\text{row total} \times \text{column total}}{\text{grand total}}$$

The expected frequency for each cell can be calculated using a 2×2 table as follows:

cell a: $[(a + b) \times (a + c)/\text{total}]$
cell b: $[(a + b) \times (b + d)/\text{total}]$
cell c: $[(a + c) \times (c + d)/\text{total}]$
cell d: $[(b + d) \times (c + d)/\text{total}]$

These are then compared using this formula, to produce the χ^2 statistic:

$$\chi^2 = \sum \frac{(O - E)^2}{E}$$

where O = observed frequencies and E = expected frequencies. Degrees of freedom (d.f.) are calculated using the following formula:

$$\text{d.f.} = (r - 1) \times (c - 1)$$

where r = number of rows and c = number of columns.

The greater the difference between the observed and expected frequencies, the less likely it is that the null hypothesis is true.

The Chi-squared test only works when **frequencies** are used in the cells. Data such as proportions, means or physical measurements are not valid. This test is used to detect an **association** between data in rows and data in columns, but it does not indicate the **strength** of any association. The Chi-squared test is more accurate when large frequencies are used – all of the **expected** frequencies should be more than 1, and at least 80% of the **expected** frequencies should be more than 5. If these **conditions**, called the assumptions of the test, are not met, the Chi-squared test is not valid and therefore cannot be used. If the Chi-squared test is not valid and a 2×2 table is being used, **Fisher's exact test** can sometimes be utilised (the formula for this test is not covered in this basic guide, but many computer programs will automatically calculate it if sufficiently small expected frequencies are detected within a 2×2 table). If there are more than two rows and/or columns, it may be possible to regroup the data so as to create fewer columns. Doing this will increase the cell frequencies, which may then be large enough to meet the requirements. For example, if you have four age groups (0–7, 8–14, 15–21 and 22–28 years), it might be reasonable to combine these to produce two age groups (0–14 and 15–28 years). However, regrouping data into fewer categories is a compromise, as the precision that is allowed by having so many categories will be reduced.

If the test is being carried out to detect an association between **paired** data where there are only two possible outcomes (e.g. the outcome is either success or failure **and** two different regimes are tried on the same individuals or on matched pairs), then **McNemar's Chi-squared test** should be used. This is not covered in this basic guide.

Let us look at an example using some real data, as shown in Table 20.2. A study asks whether Asians with diabetes receive worse treatment in primary care than non-Asians with diabetes. This is important, since Asians are more likely to develop diabetes than non-Asians. A number of variables are studied, including whether patients with diabetes have received a HbA1$_c$ test within the previous year (we mentioned HbA1$_c$ in Chapter 7), as this is a valuable indicator of how successfully diabetes is being controlled. Having the test performed regularly is important, and is therefore a valid indicator of healthcare quality in diabetes. We can calculate that 64.6% (128/198) of Asians received the check, compared with 74.7% (430/576) of non-Asians. As such we know that a lower proportion of Asian patients was checked, but is there a significant association between ethnicity and receiving the check? Our null hypothesis is that there is **no association** between ethnicity and receiving a HbA1$_c$ check.

TABLE 20.2 Frequencies for HbA1$_c$ testing by ethnic group. Adapted from Stewart and Rao (2000)

		HbA1$_c$ test done?		
		Yes	No	Total
Ethnicity of patient	Asian	128 (a)	70 (b)	198 (a + b)
	Non-Asian	430 (c)	146 (d)	576 (c + d)
	Total	558 (a + c)	216 (b + d)	774 (a + b + c + d)

The frequencies for Asian/non-Asian patients with diabetes are assembled in a 2 × 2 table and tabulated against the frequencies in each group of patients who have/have not received the HbA1$_c$ test, as shown in Table 20.2.

To calculate χ^2, use the following steps.

1. Work out the degrees of freedom (d.f.).
2. Work out the expected frequencies in each of cells a, b, c and d – **or more if it is a larger table**.

3. For each cell, subtract the expected frequency from the observed frequency $(O - E)$.
4. For each cell, square the result $(O - E)^2$.
5. For each cell, divide this number by the expected frequency $[(O - E)^2/E]$.
6. Add up the results for each cell – this gives you the χ^2 statistic.
7. Using the χ^2 distribution table in Appendix 1, look up the d.f. value in the left-hand column.
8. Read across this row until the nearest values to the left and right of your χ^2 statistic can be seen.
9. Your P-value will be **less than** the P-value at the top of the column to the left of your χ^2 statistic and **greater than** the P-value at the top of the column to its right. (For example, a χ^2 statistic of 6.128 with 2 d.f. falls in between 5.991 and 7.824. The nearest value to its left is 5.991; the P-value at the top of this column is 0.05. The P-value for your χ^2 statistic will therefore be **less than** 0.05, and is written $P < 0.05$. If your χ^2 statistic is 2.683 with 2 d.f., there is no column to its left, so the P-value will be **greater** than the column to its right, and is therefore > 0.2).

Using the data for the Asian diabetes study, let us work out χ^2.

1. There are two rows and two columns:

    $(r - 1) \times (c - 1) = (2 - 1) \times (2 - 1) = 1 \times 1$; so d.f. $= 1$.

2. Work out the expected frequencies for each cell (to two decimal places in this example):

    cell a: $[(a + b) \times (a + c)/\text{total}]$ $= (198 \times 558)/774$
             $= 110\,484/774 = 142.74$
    cell b: $[(a + b) \times (b + d)/\text{total}]$ $= (198 \times 216)/774$
             $= 42\,768/774 = 55.26$
    cell c: $[(a + c) \times (c + d)/\text{total}]$ $= (558 \times 576)/774$
             $= 321\,408/774 = 415.26$
    cell d: $[(b + d) \times (c + d)/\text{total}]$ $= (216 \times 576)/774$
             $= 124\,416/774 = 160.74$.

    Going back to the assumptions mentioned earlier in the chapter, it is clear that all of the expected frequencies are more than 1 and all are also more than 5. The Chi-squared test is therefore valid and it can be used.
3–5. It is helpful to construct a grid to aid the following calculations, as shown in Table 20.3.
6. The sum of all of the $(O - E^2/E)$ results is 7.32 – this is the χ^2 statistic.

7. On the χ^2 distribution table in Appendix 1, look along the row for d.f. = 1.
8. Look along the row to find the values to the left and right of the χ^2 statistic – it lies in between 6.635 and 10.827.
9. Reading up the columns for these two values shows that the corresponding P-value is less than 0.01 but greater than 0.001 – we can therefore write the P-value as $P < 0.01$.

TABLE 20.3 Grid showing calculations for the χ^2 statistic

	O	E (step 2)	(O – E) (step 3)	(O – E)² (step 4)	[(O – E)²/E] (step 5)
a	128	142.74	−14.74	217.27	1.52
b	70	55.26	14.74	217.27	3.93
c	430	415.26	14.74	217.27	0.52
d	146	160.74	−14.74	217.27	1.35
Total	774				7.32

Thus there is strong evidence to reject the null hypothesis, and we may conclude that there is an association between being Asian and receiving a HbA1$_c$ check. Asian patients are significantly less likely to receive a HbA1$_c$ check, and appear to receive a poorer quality of care in this respect.

The χ^2 formula is made more conservative by subtracting 0.5 from the product of $(O – E)$ at stage 3. We can ignore any minus numbers in the product of $(O – E)$, and it is thus written as $(|O – E|)$. This becomes $[|(O – E)| – 0.5]$, and is known as **Yates' correction** (also called a **continuity correction**). It is especially important to use this when frequencies are small. Note that Yates' correction can only be used for 2×2 tables. If Yates' correction is applied to the data shown, we obtain the following result, as shown in Table 20.4.

TABLE 20.4 Grid showing calculations for the χ^2 statistic with Yates' correction

	O	E (step 2)	[|(O – E)| – 0.5] (step 3)	[|(O – E)| – 0.5]² (step 4)	[(|(O – E)| – 0.5)²/E] (step 5)
a	128	142.74	14.24	202.78	1.42
b	70	55.26	14.24	202.78	3.67
c	430	415.26	14.24	202.78	0.49
d	146	160.74	14.24	202.78	1.26
Total	774				6.84

Thus $\chi^2 = 6.84$, which still gives a P-value of < 0.01. However, this is closer to the 0.01 value than the previous χ^2 of 7.32. The significance is therefore slightly reduced.

Chi-squared for trend can be used to test for a statistically significant trend in exposure groups which have **a meaningful order** and **two outcomes**. For example, this could apply to age groups (. . . 45–54, 55–64, 65–74, 75+) and **diagnosis of dementia** (Y/N) or **pain severity** (mild, moderate, severe) and **cessation of pain** (Y/N). The calculation of Chi-squared for trend is not covered in this basic guide.

CHAPTER 21

Statistical power and sample size

It is important to have a sample of the right size to allow a clinically relevant effect to be detected. For example, it would be a terrible waste of time and money to carry out a study, only to discover **at the end** that too few subjects had been included. On the other hand, investigators may wish to avoid studying, say, 3000 subjects if 150 would be sufficient (it may also be unethical to undertake such an unnecessarily large study).

Sample size calculations are therefore helpful and should always be done before carrying out a study.

As well as sample size, people often mention **the power of a study** or **whether a study has sufficient power**. These topics are related, and will be discussed in the next few pages.

In Chapter 14, we identified two types of error that should be recognised when interpreting a *P*-value:

- **type 1 error** – rejecting a **true** null hypothesis, and accepting a false alternative hypothesis. The probability of making a type 1 error is called **alpha** (α)
- **type 2 error** – **not** rejecting a **false** null hypothesis. The probability of making a type 2 error is called **beta** (β).

The level of significance is the probability of making a type 1 error (α), and it is usually set at 5% (0.05).

The **power** of a study is the probability of rejecting a false null hypothesis, so it is $1 - \beta$. This can be expressed as either a percentage or a proportion. Statistical power is used in the calculation of sample size. As sample size increases, so does the ability to reject a false null hypothesis. Beta is often set at 20%, so the power ($1 - \beta$) is 80% or 0.8. It is essential that a study has adequate power – this is normally considered to be at least 80% or 0.8.

The calculation of sample size takes the following into account:

- the level of significance (α)
- power ($1 - \beta$)
- the size of the smallest effect considered to be clinically important
- the standard deviation (SD) in the population (this may not actually be known, so it may have to be estimated from similar studies or from a pilot study).

Sample size and power calculations should always be performed in the planning stage of a study, where they are referred to as *a priori* **calculations** (before data are collected). If calculations are done later on, they are called *post-hoc* **calculations** (after data are collected) – this practice is not generally advised, though it is sometimes requested by reviewers when considering a study submitted for publication.

This chapter will concentrate on sample size calculations for two common situations – continuous data for two independent groups and categorical data for two independent groups. These calculations will assume that studies have two patient groups of **equal** size. Several texts present formulae and guidance for other situations not described here (*see* Further reading) and various websites are available online.

We shall avoid complicated formulae and focus instead on **Altman's nomogram** and an **internet-based sample size calculator**, then work through some examples using each method.

Both methods can be used to calculate either sample size or power.

ALTMAN'S NOMOGRAM

This is a useful device for calculating sample size or power in a variety of situations. Calculations are relatively simple and straightforward. The nomogram is shown in Figure 21.1.

Use of the nomogram requires only one calculation – the **standardised difference**. This is the ratio of the effect being studied to the relevant SD. There are different formulae for the standardised difference, according to the situation. These will be shown along with fully worked examples later in this chapter.

When the standardised difference has been calculated, the total sample size is found by using a ruler (preferably transparent) or drawing a line between the standardised difference (listed down the left-hand side of the nomogram) and the power (down the right-hand side). The total sample size is shown where the line you have made crosses the slanted 'N' line on the nomogram.

Alternatively, making a line connecting standardised difference and sample size allows the power of a study to be found.

Details of how to use the nomogram for other types of sample size and power calculations can be found in Altman (1991) and other texts.

We can try this now, using a simple example. If we have a standardised difference of 0.9, and power of 0.8, then a total sample size of around 38 will be required for a significance level of 0.05. That is, there should be 19 in each group.

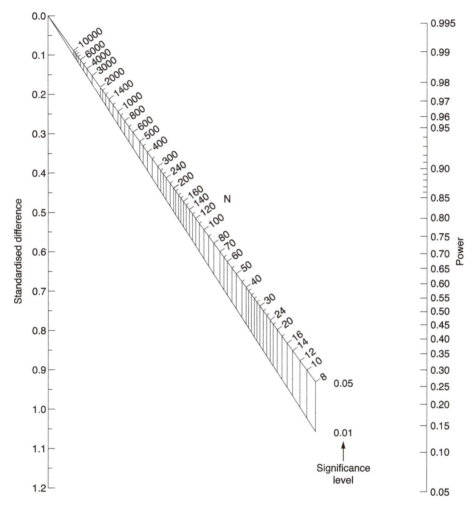

FIGURE 21.1 Altman's nomogram for calculating sample size or power (Altman, 1982) (reproduced with permission of Professor D Altman and Wiley-Blackwell).

To see the sample size for the 0.01 significance level, look at where your line crosses the '0.01' line, then draw another line upwards and read off the scale. Approximately 56 (28 in each group) will be required – see the vertical line, shown in Figure 21.2.

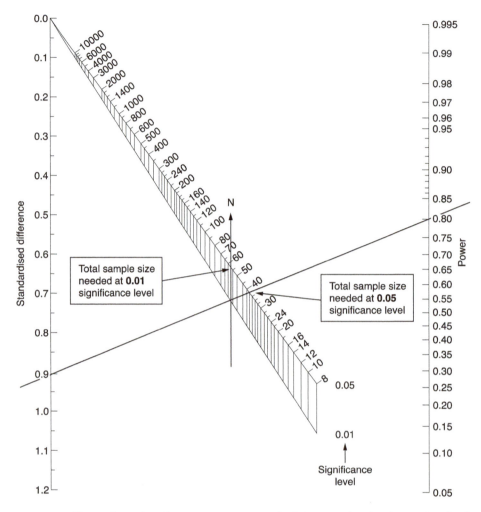

FIGURE 21.2 Example, using the nomogram to calculate sample size for a standardised difference of 0.9, and power of 0.8 (reproduced with permission of Professor D Altman and Wiley-Blackwell).

We shall work through more examples later.

We can also use the nomogram to calculate the **power** of a study. With a standardised difference of 0.8 and a total sample size of 65, the power is approximately 0.9. This is shown in Figure 21.3.

This is sometimes performed after a study has been completed – especially when no sample size calculation was originally done – and when this is the case, it is called a 'post-hoc' power calculation.

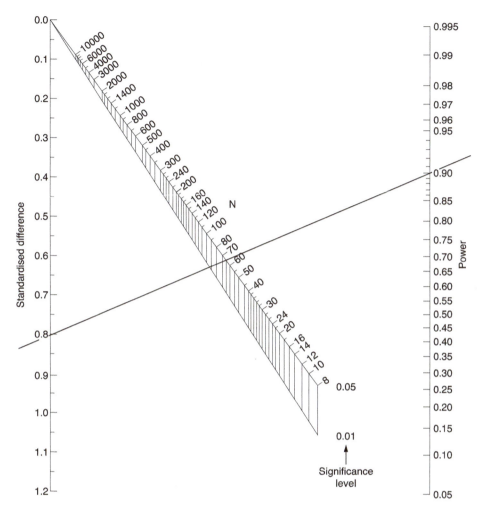

FIGURE 21.3 Example, using the nomogram to calculate power for a standardised difference of 0.8, and total sample size of 65 (reproduced with permission of Professor D Altman and Wiley-Blackwell).

COMPUTERISED SAMPLE SIZE CALCULATIONS

A quick internet search will reveal many online sample size and power calculators. Some can be downloaded and saved for installation and use offline, while others are exclusively online tools. It is difficult to recommend just one, but Professor Rollin Brant at the University of British Columbia has developed an online calculator that is very accessible, free and easy to use. The calculator is available at www.stat.ubc. ca/~rollin/stats/ssize/

After connecting to the site, just click on one of the five options shown. After entering the required details, the sample size will be displayed.

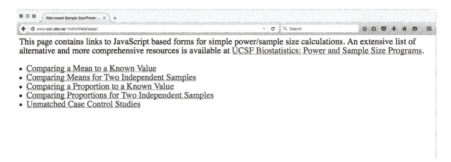

FIGURE 21.4 Opening screen for online sample size calculator (reproduced with permission of Professor Rollin Brant).

For example, if we want to find the sample size for a study where independent *t*-tests will be used for data analysis, click on the second option 'Comparing Means for Two Independent Samples'. *See* Figure 21.5.

Inference for Means: Comparing Two Independent Samples

(To use this page, your browser must recognize JavaScript.)

Choose which calculation you desire, enter the relevant population values for mu1 (mean of population 1), mu2 (mean of population 2), and sigma (common standard deviation) and, if calculating power, a sample size (assumed the same for each sample). You may also modify α (type I error rate) and the power, if relevant. After making your entries, hit the calculate button at the bottom.

- Calculate Sample Size (for specified Power)
- Calculate Power (for specified Sample Size)

Enter a value for mu1:
Enter a value for mu2:
Enter a value for sigma:

- 1 Sided Test
- 2 Sided Test

Enter a value for α (default is .05): .05
Enter a value for desired power (default is .80): .80
The sample size (for each sample separately) is:

Calculate

Reference: The calculations are the customary ones based on normal distributions. See for example *Hypothesis Testing: Two-Sample Inference - Estimation of Sample Size and Power for Comparing Two Means* in Bernard Rosner's **Fundamentals of Biostatistics**.

Rollin Brant
Email me at: rollin@stat.ubc.ca

FIGURE 21.5 Data entry screen for 'Comparing Means for Two Independent Samples'.

The program assumes that we want to calculate sample size for two-sided tests, with a significant level of 0.05 and a power of 0.8. These fields can either be left unchanged, or overwritten as required. Power can be calculated, rather than sample size, by clicking 'Calculate Power', instead of 'Calculate Sample Size'.

Imagine we are planning a study to detect a clinically important reduction from 50 to 45 units, with a population SD of 6.9 (shown in Figure 21.6).

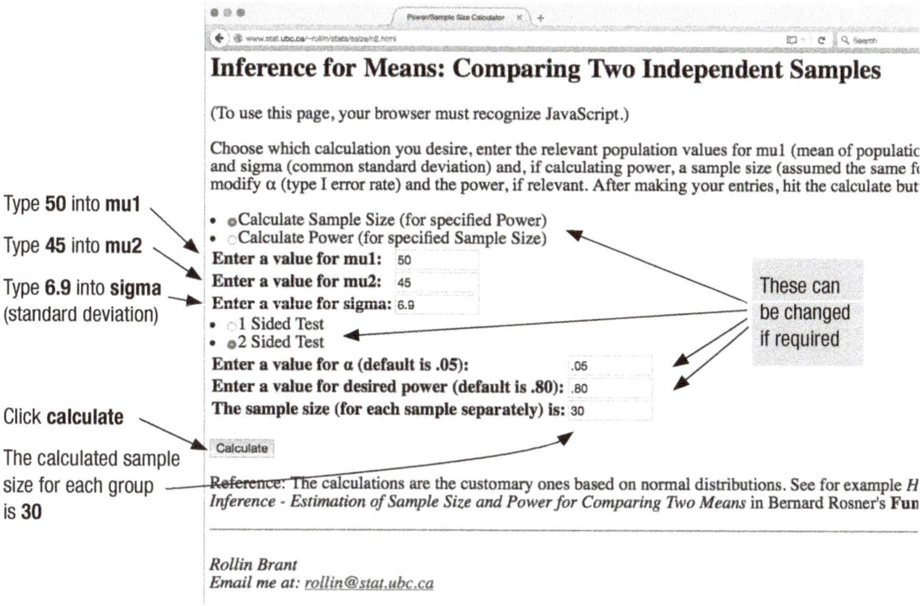

Type **50** into **mu1**

Type **45** into **mu2**

Type **6.9** into **sigma** (standard deviation)

Click **calculate**

The calculated sample size for each group is **30**

Inference for Means: Comparing Two Independent Samples

(To use this page, your browser must recognize JavaScript.)

Choose which calculation you desire, enter the relevant population values for mu1 (mean of populatic and sigma (common standard deviation) and, if calculating power, a sample size (assumed the same fo modify α (type I error rate) and the power, if relevant. After making your entries, hit the calculate but

- ⊙ Calculate Sample Size (for specified Power)
- ○ Calculate Power (for specified Sample Size)

Enter a value for mu1: 50
Enter a value for mu2: 45
Enter a value for sigma: 6.9
- ○ 1 Sided Test
- ⊙ 2 Sided Test

Enter a value for α (default is .05): .05
Enter a value for desired power (default is .80): .80
The sample size (for each sample separately) is: 30

Calculate

These can be changed if required

Reference: The calculations are the customary ones based on normal distributions. See for example *H Inference - Estimation of Sample Size and Power for Comparing Two Means* in Bernard Rosner's **Fun**

Rollin Brant
Email me at: rollin@stat.ubc.ca

FIGURE 21.6 Completed data entry screen for 'Comparing Means for Two Independent Samples'.

We will now use the nomogram and computerised methods to perform two further sample size calculations.

EXAMPLE 1: MEANS – COMPARING TWO INDEPENDENT SAMPLES

You are planning to evaluate a new treatment for delirium. The aim of the treatment is to reduce the number of days that delirium patients need to spend in hospital. Statistical analysis will use independent *t*-tests for two independent groups (patients receiving the new treatment vs. current treatment). A published paper states that the best current treatment results in a mean hospital stay of 20.5 days, and has an SD of 7.2. You and your colleagues agree that the smallest effect considered to be clinically important is **a reduction of 5 days** – to a mean of 15.5 days in hospital.

Using Altman's nomogram

The first step is to calculate the standardised difference. This is the effect being studied (reduction in number of days' stay), divided by the SD. The standardised difference is thus calculated as: $5/7.2 = \mathbf{0.69}$. We want to use a significance level of **0.05**, and power of **0.8**.

To find the sample size on the nomogram:

- make a line from 0.69 on the standardised difference line (down the left-hand side) to 0.8 on the power line (down the right-hand side)
- read off the total sample size along the 0.05 significance level line.

As shown in Figure 21.7, this crosses the 0.05 line at approximately 65, indicating that around 32 patients will be needed for each group.

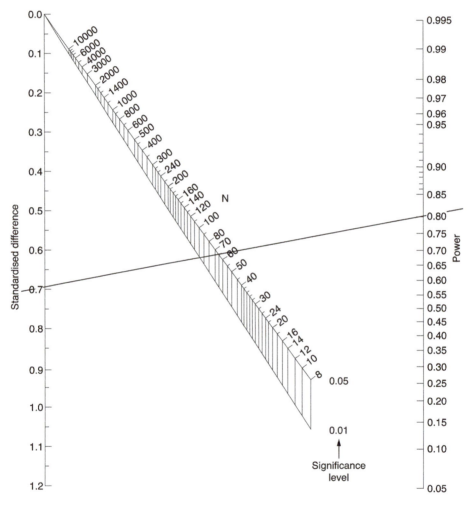

FIGURE 21.7 Nomogram, showing total sample size required for delirium study (reproduced with permission of Professor D Altman and Wiley-Blackwell).

Using the online calculator

After accessing the online sample size calculator, select the second option 'Comparing Means for Two Independent Samples':

- type in the mean days' hospital stay (with current treatment) into **mu1** – 20.5
- type in the mean days' hospital stay (expected with new treatment) into **mu2** – 15.5
- type the SD into **sigma** – 7.2
- click 'Calculate'
- the sample size for each group is **33**.

This is shown in Figure 21.8. You can see that the two methods produce nearly identical results. The nomogram does not require access to a computer, but precision depends on how accurately the line is made.

EXAMPLE 2: PROPORTIONS – COMPARING TWO INDEPENDENT SAMPLES

This study plans to compare the effectiveness of two psychological treatments for anxiety. It is anticipated that the new treatment will be more effective than the current treatment. Statistical analysis will use the Chi-squared test for association between effectiveness and the two independent groups (complete relief from anxiety in patients receiving the new treatment vs. current treatment). A paper in a peer-reviewed journal reports that the best current treatment produces complete relief from anxiety in 30% (or 0.3, as a proportion) of cases. You agree that the smallest effect considered to be clinically important is complete relief in 40% (or 0.4, as a proportion) of cases. Note that it is essential that we work with proportions here, not percentages.

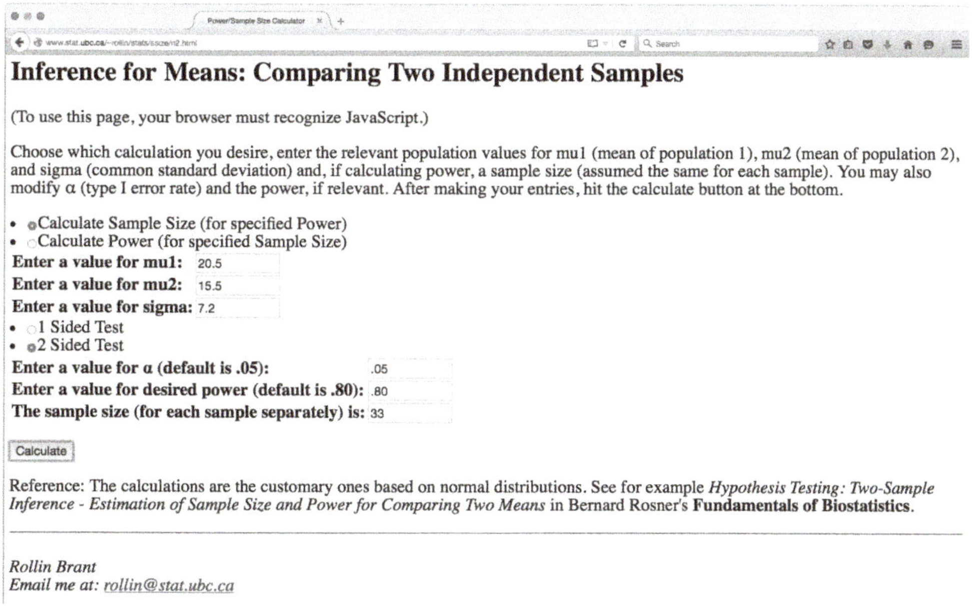

Inference for Means: Comparing Two Independent Samples

(To use this page, your browser must recognize JavaScript.)

Choose which calculation you desire, enter the relevant population values for mu1 (mean of population 1), mu2 (mean of population 2), and sigma (common standard deviation) and, if calculating power, a sample size (assumed the same for each sample). You may also modify α (type I error rate) and the power, if relevant. After making your entries, hit the calculate button at the bottom.

- ⊙ Calculate Sample Size (for specified Power)
- ○ Calculate Power (for specified Sample Size)

Enter a value for mu1: 20.5
Enter a value for mu2: 15.5
Enter a value for sigma: 7.2
- ○ 1 Sided Test
- ⊙ 2 Sided Test

Enter a value for α (default is .05): .05
Enter a value for desired power (default is .80): .80
The sample size (for each sample separately) is: 33

[Calculate]

Reference: The calculations are the customary ones based on normal distributions. See for example *Hypothesis Testing: Two-Sample Inference - Estimation of Sample Size and Power for Comparing Two Means* in Bernard Rosner's **Fundamentals of Biostatistics**.

Rollin Brant
Email me at: rollin@stat.ubc.ca

FIGURE 21.8 Completed data entry screen, showing total sample size required for delirium study.

Using Altman's nomogram

Calculating the **standardised difference** is a little more complex here, but is fairly straightforward to work through. The formula is:

$$\frac{p_1 - p_2}{\sqrt{\bar{p}(1-\bar{p})}}$$

where $\bar{p} = (p_1 + p_2)/2$

p refers to proportions

$p_1 = 0.4$ and $p_2 = 0.3$

$\bar{p} = (0.4 + 0.3)/2 = \bar{p} = (0.7)/2 = \bar{p} = 0.35$

The standardised difference is therefore calculated as:

$$\frac{0.4 - 0.3}{\sqrt{0.35(1-0.35)}} = \frac{0.1}{\sqrt{0.35(1-0.35)}} = \frac{0.1}{\sqrt{0.35(0.65)}}$$

$$= \frac{0.1}{\sqrt{0.2275}} = \frac{0.1}{0.4769696} = 0.2097 \text{ or } 0.21$$

(the above is correct to 2 decimal places)

For this study, we will use a significance level of **0.01**, and power of **0.8**. To find the sample size on the nomogram:

- make a line from 0.21 on the standardised difference line (down the left-hand side) to 0.8 on the power line (down the right-hand side)
- read off the total sample size along the 0.01 significance level line (follow the vertical line up from the 0.01 line and read off the numbered scale).

As shown in Figure 21.9, this crosses the 0.01 line at approximately 1050, indicating that around 525 patients will be needed for each group.

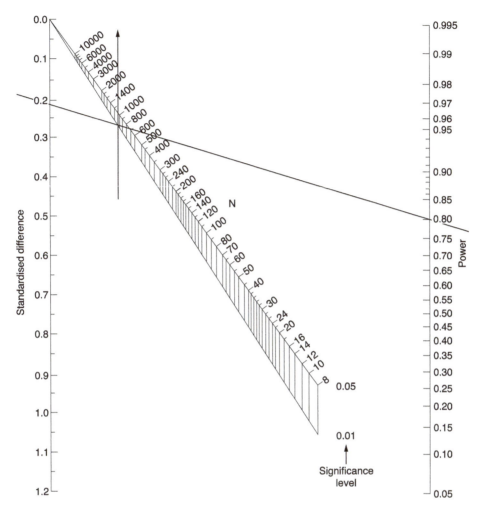

FIGURE 21.9 Nomogram, showing total sample size required for anxiety study (reproduced with permission of Professor D Altman and Wiley-Blackwell).

Using the online calculator

After accessing the online sample size calculator, select the fourth option 'Comparing Proportions for Two Independent Samples':

- type in the proportion of complete relief from anxiety (expected, with the new treatment) into *p1* – 0.4
- type in the proportion of complete relief from anxiety (with current treatment) into *p2* – 0.3
- change the value for α to 0.01

- click 'Calculate'
- the sample size for each group is **530**.

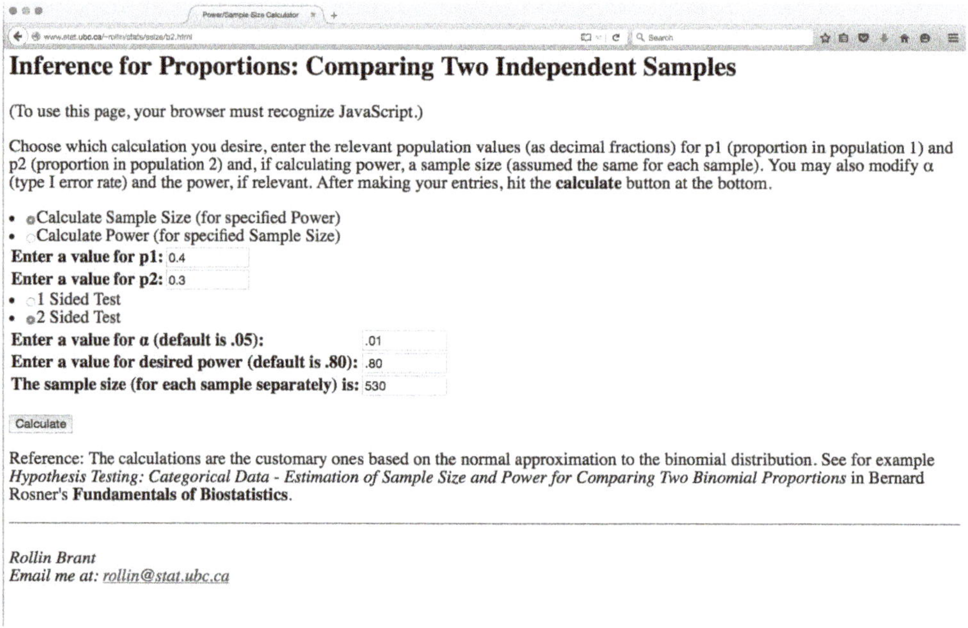

FIGURE 21.10 Completed data entry screen, showing total sample size required for anxiety study.

CHAPTER 22

Effect size

We have so far discussed the role of *P*-values and the useful extra information that confidence intervals can supply. *P*-values tell us whether there is statistical significance, and a 95% confidence interval is the interval which includes the true population mean value in 95% of cases.

When we are looking at the difference between two mean values, however, neither the *P*-value nor the confidence interval tells us whether the **size** of this difference is practically meaningful.

Something that can be helpful with this is the **effect size**. Essentially, this is the size of the difference in mean values between two groups, relative to the standard deviation (SD) (Barton & Peat, 2014).

One commonly used measure of effect size is **Cohen's *d***. For **two independent groups**, its calculation involves dividing the difference between the two means by the SD (there are different ways of calculating Cohen's *d* for other situations):

$$\text{Effect size} = d = \frac{m_1 - m_2}{SD}$$

where: m_1 = mean of sample 1, m_2 = mean of sample 2 and SD = standard deviation

Note: only the **difference** between the two means is important, so any minus numbers can be ignored.

It is good practice to report effect sizes as you would with *P*-values, confidence intervals, etc.

The formula looks quite straightforward, but how do we get **one** SD for two separate samples? In the unlikely event that both samples have the same SD, that value can be used. If the mean values have different SDs and there is either a baseline measurement or a control group, we should use the SD of the baseline/control group. If there is no baseline/control group, then a pooled SD can be used, calculated in this situation as follows:

$$\text{Pooled SD} = \sqrt{\frac{(SD_1^2 + SD_2^2)}{2}}$$

where: SD_1 is the standard deviation of mean 1, and SD_2 is the standard deviation of mean 2.

Having said this, **Cohen's *d*** is most reliable when sample size and SD are equal in both groups. In any event, data should be (at least approximately) normally distributed.

When using Cohen's *d*, an effect size of 0.2 is regarded as small, 0.5 medium and 0.8 large (Cohen, 1988). The value of Cohen's *d* can extend beyond 1.0.

As you can see, the calculation of effect size is relatively simple, so let's have a go at working through an example.

> A study evaluated two psychological therapies, with the aim of increasing mental well-being. The mental well-being of 60 patients treated with a course of a new therapy (group 1) was compared with that of a control group of 60 further patients who had received a course of a standard therapy (group 2). The Warwick-Edinburgh Mental Well-being Scale (NHS Health Scotland, University of Warwick and University of Edinburgh*, 2006) instrument was used to measure mental well-being in both groups. The WEMWBS produces a score of between 14 and 70; the higher the score, the higher the well-being.
>
> At the end of treatment, the study found that in group 1, the mean score was 45.78 (SD = 12.95) and in group 2 the mean score was 37.23 (SD = 11.24). An independent *t*-test was carried out, and the difference in mean scores was significant (d.f. = 118, $t = -7.407$, $P < 0.001$).
>
> It is therefore apparent that mean mental well-being scores at the end of treatment were higher in patients receiving the new therapy compared with standard therapy, and the difference was statistically significant. But how large was the size of the treatment effect?
>
> We know that the formula for Cohen's *d* is: $\frac{m_1 - m_2}{SD}$
>
> We also know that m_1 (mean score of group 1) = 45.78 and m_2 (mean score of group 2) = 37.23
>
> For SD, we could use the SD of the control group (group 2) of 11.24, and can now complete our effect size calculation:

$$d = \frac{m_1 - m_2}{SD}$$

$$= \frac{45.78 - 37.23}{SD}$$

$$= \frac{8.55}{SD}$$

$$= \frac{8.55}{11.24}$$

= **0.76** – a medium to large effect size.

We can therefore report that in this study, the mean mental well-being score at the end of treatment was 45.78 (SD = 12.95) in patients receiving the new therapy, compared with 37.23 (SD = 11.24) in those receiving the standard therapy; this difference was significant (d.f. = 118, t = –7.407) with a medium to large effect size (d = 0.76).

It should be noted that in this study, the 'medium' effect size was very close to a 'large' effect size. Effect size classification should be interpreted as a guide only and treated accordingly. A difference of 8.55 in WEMWBS scores for this patient group may be regarded as 'medium' according to the Cohen's d classification, but this does not necessarily mean it would be considered as a 'medium' effect in any **clinical** sense. On the other hand, because Cohen's d is a standardised measurement of effect size, we can usefully compare effect sizes between other similar studies that report Cohen's d. It is also important to remember that effect size is not influenced by sample size – so a very small study could have a 'large' effect size, which would provide little reliable evidence.

Shall we have a go at calculating a pooled SD? Let's see how much difference it would make to the effect size calculation just given if we used a pooled SD instead of the control group SD. We will use the two SDs (12.95 and 11.24) from the before and after therapy mean WEMWBS scores, as reported.

$$\text{Pooled } SD = \sqrt{\frac{(SD_1^2 + SD_2^2)}{2}}$$

$$= \sqrt{\frac{(12.95^2 + 11.24^2)}{2}}$$

$$= \sqrt{\frac{(167.70 + 126.34)}{2}}$$

$$= \sqrt{\frac{294.04}{2}}$$

$$= \sqrt{147.02}$$

$$= \mathbf{12.13}$$

To complete our effect size calculation using pooled SD:

$$d = \frac{m_1 - m_2}{SD}$$

$$= \frac{45.78 - 37.23}{SD}$$

$$= \frac{8.55}{SD}$$

$$= \frac{8.55}{12.13}$$

$$= 0.7049 \text{ or } \mathbf{0.70} \text{ to two decimal places.}$$

Going back to our classification of d, 0.70 would be a medium to large effect size. This is slightly smaller than the effect size calculated using the control group SD because the scores of group 1 are rather more variable (i.e. the SD is larger).

As mentioned earlier, there are different methods for calculating Cohen's d in other situations (e.g. for a paired t-test), which are not covered by this basic guide. There are also other measures of effect size in addition to Cohen's d. Please see other sources or consult a statistician if more detail is required.

In the first half of this book, we have discussed the main types of data and basic statistical analysis that are used in healthcare. If there is anything that you are unsure about, now might be a good time to go back and re-read the particular section in which it appears.

If you are ready to continue, the second half of the book deals with epidemiology. Here we shall explore a range of methods, including those that will help you to measure the amount of disease in groups of people, to search for possible causes of disease and death, and to try to improve survival by undertaking screening to identify an illness before the symptoms even develop.

CHAPTER 23

What is epidemiology?

Epidemiology is the study of how often diseases occur in different groups of people, and why (Coggon *et al.*, 1997). Medicine often asks 'Why has this person got this disease?' and 'What is the best way of treating them?'. However, epidemiology asks broader questions such as 'What kind of people get this disease?', 'Why do they get it when others don't?' and 'How can we find out what is generally the best way of treating people with this disease?' (Department of Public Health and Epidemiology, 1999).

Epidemiology can be used to formulate strategies for managing established illness, as well as for preventing further cases. An epidemiological investigation will usually involve the selection of a **sample** from a **population**. This is discussed in Chapters 2 and 3.

People who have a disease or condition that is being studied are generally referred to as **cases**. People without the disease are called **non-cases**. Epidemiological studies known as **case–control studies** (*see* Chapter 30) compare groups of cases with non-cases. **Cohort studies** (*see* Chapter 29) compare groups of people who have been **exposed** to a particular **risk factor** for a disease with other groups who have not been exposed in this way. When these types of comparisons are made, the non-cases or non-exposed individuals are referred to as **controls**. In these types of study, the groups are called **study groups**.

Randomised controlled trials (*see* Chapter 31) often compare a group of people who are receiving a certain treatment with another group who are receiving a different treatment or even a 'dummy' treatment called a **placebo**. In randomised controlled trials, the groups are usually called **treatment arms**.

A number of techniques exist for measuring disease and evaluating results. Some of these are explained in this basic guide, together with definitions of a range of epidemiological terms.

CHAPTER 24

Bias and confounding

BIAS

Epidemiological studies try to provide accurate answers to questions such as 'What is the prevalence of smoking in this district's population?' or 'What is the additional risk of liver cancer due to previous hepatitis B infection?'. It is almost certain that the estimates which are obtained are different to the **real** prevalence or the **real** risk. This error in estimating the true effect is caused by two sources of error – **random** and **systematic** error. Random errors will always occur from time to time (e.g. an investigator records a temperature measurement incorrectly, or allocates a patient to treatment group A when they were supposed to be in treatment group B), but have no particular pattern. Systematic errors happen when the errors are arising more uniformly (e.g. a certain investigator's temperature readings are regularly higher than those made by other investigators, or the mean age of patients in one treatment group is considerably higher than that in another group). Features of a study that produce systematic error are generally referred to as **bias**.

Bias is an undesirable feature of study design that tends to produce results which are **systematically** different from the real values. It can apply to all types of study, and it usually occurs due to faults in the way in which a study is planned and carried out. In some circumstances, bias can make the results of a study completely unreliable.

It is very difficult to avoid bias completely. However, it is possible to limit any problems by seeking out and eliminating potential biases as early as possible. The ideal time to do this is during the planning stages of a study. If detected at a later stage, biases can sometimes (but not always) be reduced by taking them into account during data analysis and interpretation. In particular, studies should be scrutinised to detect bias. Errors in **data analysis** can also produce bias, and should be similarly sought out and dealt with. The main types of bias are **selection bias** and **information bias**.

Selection bias

Selection bias occurs as a result of errors in identifying the study population. It can occur due to factors such as the following.

- Systematically excluding or over-representing certain groups – this is called **sampling bias**. For example, a study designed to estimate the prevalence of smoking in a population may select subjects for interview in a number of locations, including a city centre. If the interviews are only conducted on weekdays, the study is likely to under-represent people who are in full-time employment, and to include a higher proportion of those who are unemployed, off work or mothers with children.
- Systematic differences in the way in which subjects are recruited into different groups for a study – this is called **allocation bias**. For example, a study may fail to use random sampling – the first 20 patients who arrive at a clinic are allocated to a new treatment, and the next 20 patients are allocated to an existing treatment. However, the patients who arrive early may be fitter or wealthier, or alternatively the doctor may have asked to see the most seriously ill patients first.
- Missed responders or non-responders – this is called **responder bias**. For example, a study may send questionnaires to members of the control group. If these subjects are from a different social class to the cases, there may be differences in the proportion of responses that are received. Furthermore, controls who are non-cases may see little point in responding.

Information bias

This is caused by systematic differences in data collection, measurement or classification. Some common causes of information bias include the following.

- People suffering from a disease may have spent more time thinking of possible links between their past behaviour and their disease than non-sufferers – this is known as **recall bias**. It may result in systematic differences between cases and controls. Cases may therefore report more exposure to possible hazards.
- Some subjects may exaggerate or understate their responses, or deny that they engage in embarrassing or undesirable activities – this is called **social acceptability bias**.
- Medical records may contain more information on patients who are 'cases' – this is called **recording bias**.
- Interviewers may phrase questions differently for different subjects, or write down their own interpretations of what subjects have said – this is called **interviewer bias**.
- In studies that follow up subjects at intervals, people from certain groups may tend to be lost to follow-up, or a disproportionate number of exposed subjects may be

lost to follow-up compared with non-exposed subjects – this is called **follow-up bias**.

- Patients may be systematically misclassified as either having disease or exposure, and will thus produce **misclassification bias**.
- Some groups may give different responses. For example, older people of lower social class may be less likely to express dissatisfaction with a health-related service.
- Investigators may look more closely at exposed patients, to try to find the presence of a disease, or they may be more attentive to certain types of subjects.

CONFOUNDING

Confounding occurs when a separate factor (or factors) influences the risk of developing a disease, other than the risk factor being studied. To be a confounder, the factor has to be related to the exposure, and it also has to be an independent risk factor for the disease being studied.

For example, if a study assesses whether high alcohol consumption is a risk factor for coronary heart disease, smoking is a **confounding factor** (also called a **confounder**) (*see* Figure 24.1). This is because smoking is known to be related to alcohol consumption, and it is also a risk factor for coronary heart disease.

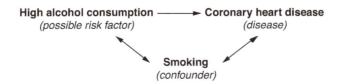

FIGURE 24.1 An example of confounding. After Lilienfeld and Stolley (1994).

Age and sex are also common causes of confounding, as well as factors such as ethnicity and smoking. For example, we know that mortality is higher in older people, men tend to die earlier than women, African-Caribbean people are at increased risk of developing hypertension and people who smoke are much more likely than non-smokers to develop diseases such as lung cancer and coronary heart disease.

The best way to deal with a possible confounding factor is to eliminate its effect from the study. Methods to achieve this include the following.

- **Randomisation** – ensuring that samples are randomly selected (*see* Chapter 3).
- **Matching** – in case–control studies (*see* Chapter 30), controls are matched to cases at the start of the study according to particular characteristics which are known to be present in cases (e.g. age, sex, smoking, ethnic group, etc.).
- **Stratified analysis** – dividing subjects into groups at the analysis stage (e.g. by sex,

age group, smokers/non-smokers) and analysing on this basis. In the mentioned study on high alcohol consumption and coronary heart disease, it would be important to ascertain whether heavy drinkers who **also smoke** are more likely to develop coronary heart disease. An excess of coronary heart disease among this group of heavy drinkers **and** smokers would indicate that smoking is acting as a confounder.

CHAPTER 25

Measuring disease frequency

As stated previously, people who **have a disease or condition being studied** are generally referred to as **cases**. People **without the disease** are called **non-cases**. The terms **mortality** and **morbidity** are also used in many epidemiological studies. **Mortality** refers to death from a disease. **Morbidity** means the situation of living with a disease, and it is often measured in terms of **incidence** and **prevalence**. It is important to distinguish between these two terms, which are often used incorrectly.

INCIDENCE

This is the number of **new** cases in a particular time period. For example, the 'incidence of lung cancer during 2009' means the number of newly diagnosed cases of lung cancer during that year. It is calculated as follows:

$$\frac{\text{number of new cases in a given time period}}{\text{person years at risk during same time period}}$$

Person years at risk means the total amount of time (in years) that each member of the population being studied (**study population**) is at risk of the disease during the period of interest. In practice, we often do not know the exact number of person years at risk, so a proxy measure such as the mid-year population or total list size can be used.

PREVALENCE

This is defined as the proportion of current cases in a population at a given point in time. For example, the prevalence of angina in the UK is the proportion of people in the UK who are currently living with diagnosed angina. It is usually called the **point prevalence**, and is calculated as follows:

$$\frac{\text{number of cases in the population at a given point in time}}{\text{total population at the same point in time}}$$

Rates of incidence, prevalence and mortality are sometimes described as **crude** or **specific**.

CRUDE RATES

The **crude rate** refers to the number of occurrences for a whole population. It is often expressed as a rate per 1000 members of the population, but can be expressed per 10 000 or per 100 000 – for example, 'The total annual death rate in town X was 11 per 1000'. This is convenient, since there is only one figure to deal with.

To calculate a **crude death rate**, simply divide the number of deaths in a given time period by the number in the population in the same time period, and then multiply the result by 1000 (for rates per 1000) or 100 000 (for rates per 100 000), etc. If the time period is a particular year (e.g. 2012), then the mid-year population estimate should be used. Some examples of crude death rates, and their calculation are shown in Table 25.1.

However, with regard to crude rates it should be remembered that each population is likely to have a different age/sex structure. Therefore crude death rates should not be used for making like-for-like comparisons between populations.

TABLE 25.1 Grid showing calculations for crude death rates

Example	Number of deaths (a)	Population (b)	Crude death rate (to four decimal places)	Crude death rate per 100 000 (a/b) × 100 000
1	18	2300	0.0078	780
2	2	8600	0.0002	20
3	16	18 800	0.0009	90
4	14	22 300	0.0006	60
5	46	26 700	0.0017	170

SPECIFIC RATES

It is often more beneficial to subdivide crude rates into **specific rates** for age and sex. This is especially useful because the occurrence of many diseases varies with age and sex.

Specific rates can take the form of sex-specific rates (giving rates for males and females separately) or age-specific (quoting rates in specific age bands, e.g. 0–4, 5–14, 15–24 years, etc.) or age/sex-specific rates (e.g. giving rates for males aged 0–4 and

5–14 years, etc. and females aged 0–4 and 5–14 years, etc). Although these rates provide more information than crude rates, they are more onerous to evaluate because it is necessary to compare each group. This is especially problematic if there are many groups.

For specific rates, a crude rate is calculated for each group, allowing the rates for each group to be compared.

In the example shown in Table 25.2, **age-specific** death rates are calculated for deaths of children in three age groups. It is immediately obvious that there are more deaths in the < 1 year group. This would not have been apparent from crude rates alone. Indeed, the **overall** crude death rate for this group of children is 170 per 100 000, as shown in example 5 in Table 25.1.

The incidence of lung cancer increases with age, and men are generally at higher risk than women. A comparison of crude lung cancer incidence rates may indicate little change over a period of 30 years. However, by using age- and sex-specific rates it might be found that the incidence of lung cancer is decreasing in younger men, while it is increasing in older women. This might prompt further investigation into the underlying reasons for these differences.

TABLE 25.2 Grid showing calculations for age-specific death rates

Age group (years)	Number of deaths (a)	Population (b)	Crude death rate (to four decimal places)	Crude death rate per 100 000 (a/b) × 100 000
<1	25	2476	0.0101	1010
1–4	17	7523	0.0023	230
5–14	4	16 701	0.0002	20
Total	46	26 700		

As a further example, it was discovered that crude mortality rates for two seaside towns were very different. These rates were higher in Bournemouth than in Southampton. This might have suggested that Bournemouth was a more unhealthy place in which to live. However, when the deaths were divided into age-specific groups, it became evident that more people in Bournemouth died after the age of 65 years. Further investigation revealed that Bournemouth contained a higher proportion of pensioners and was often used as a place of retirement. The excess deaths could therefore be attributed to the more elderly population in Bournemouth, rather than to any 'unhealthy' factors (Coggon *et al.*, 1997).

STANDARDISATION

As was discussed earlier, it can be unwise to draw firm conclusions from crude rates. Specific rates can provide more accurate and meaningful data, but the results are time-consuming to interpret. One way of overcoming this problem is to use a **standardised rate**. This adjusts for differences in age and sex structures between the populations, allowing straightforward comparisons to be made. Although age is normally used in this process, other factors (e.g. ethnic group, etc.) can also be employed. A single statistic is produced, allowing comparisons between populations to be made easily.

Standardisation can be calculated using either **direct** or **indirect** methods. Both compare a specific study population with a 'standard population' (often England and Wales, although other populations can be used). This is usually carried out for one sex only, or for both sexes individually.

Direct standardisation

In this method, the number of deaths per 10 000 (or per 1000, per 100 000, etc.) for each group in the study population is multiplied by the proportion of individuals in each age group within the standard population. This produces the **expected** number of deaths that would have been experienced by the standard population if it had the same death rate as the study population. The resulting values for each age group are then added together to produce an **age-standardised death rate** per 10 000.

Let us work through the fictional example shown in Table 25.3.

TABLE 25.3 Mortality from bowel cancer in women aged 50–65 years, during 2010 in Mediwell

Age group (years)	Bowel cancer deaths per 10 000 women in Mediwell (A)	Proportion of women aged 50–65 years in standard population (B)	Expected deaths (A × B)
50–55	4.1	0.381	1.562
56–60	8.5	0.332	2.822
61–65	28.4	0.287	8.151
Total			12.535

The following steps can be used.

1. For each age group, multiply the number of deaths per 10 000 in the study population (A) by the proportion in the standard population (B). This gives the expected number of deaths (A × B) for each age group
2. Add up the expected deaths. This is the standardised death rate per 10 000.

Using the data in Table 25.3, we can work out the age-standardised death rate per 10 000 for women aged between 50 and 65 years in Mediwell.

1. For each age group, multiply the number of bowel cancer deaths per 10 000 (A) by the proportion of women in the standard population (B). The result is shown in the 'A × B' column, and is the expected number of deaths.
2. Add up the expected deaths to obtain the age-standardised death rate per 10 000 – this is **12.535**.

This figure could be compared with an age-standardised death rate in another area. The neighbouring town of Stediwell may have an age-standardised death rate of 15.6 per 10 000 for bowel cancer deaths in women aged 50–65 years. It is clear that Mediwell has the lower age-standardised rate.

Age-standardised rates for particular local populations can be directly compared with each other. However, it should be remembered that age-specific rates are not always available for local populations, and may in any case be too small to allow accurate estimates to be made.

Indirect standardisation

This is the most commonly used method. It yields more stable results than direct standardisation for small populations or small numbers of events. The figure produced by this method is called the **standardised mortality ratio** or **SMR**.

Death rates for age groups (or other groups) in the standard population are multiplied by the population of the same groups in the study population. This produces an 'expected' number of deaths representing what the number of deaths in the study population would have been, if that population had the same death rates as the standard population. The observed (or actual) number of deaths in the study population is then divided by the total expected number and multiplied by 100. This produces an SMR. The standard population always has an SMR of 100, with which the SMR of the study population can be compared. The SMR figure is actually a percentage. This means that if the study population's SMR is 130, its death rate is 30% higher than that of the standard population. If the study population's SMR is 86, then its death rate is 14% lower than that of the standard population.

At this point, it may be helpful to try a worked example of SMR calculation, as shown in Table 25.4.

The formula for calculating an SMR is:

$$\text{SMR} = \frac{\text{observed deaths}}{\text{expected deaths}} \times 100$$

The stages involved in calculating an SMR are as follows:

1. For each age group, multiply the death rates in the standard population (A) by the number of subjects in the study population (B), and call the result A × B. This gives the number of expected deaths in the study population.
2. Add up the expected deaths and call this result E.
3. Add up all of the observed deaths in the study population and call this result O.
4. Divide the total number of observed deaths (O) by the total number of expected deaths (E).
5. Multiply the result of O/E by 100 to obtain the SMR.

TABLE 25.4 Mortality from all causes in men aged 30–59 years, during 2011

Age group (years)	Observed deaths in Mediwell	Death rates for males in the standard population (A)	Population of males aged 30–59 years in Mediwell (B)	Expected deaths of males in Mediwell, based on males in standard population (A × B)
30–39	34	0.00096	27 000	25.92
40–49	82	0.0027	24 700	66.69
50–59	171	0.0072	21 400	154.08
Total	287 (O)			246.69 (E)

To calculate the SMR for deaths in men aged 30–59 years in Mediwell, the following steps are involved.

1. For each age group, multiply the death rates in the standard population (A) by the number of subjects in the study population (B) to obtain the number of expected deaths in the study population. The result is shown in the 'A × B' column of Table 25.4.
2. Add up the expected deaths. The total number is 246.69 (E).
3. Add up all of the observed deaths in the study population. The total number is 287 (O).
4. Divide the total number of observed deaths (O) by the total number of expected deaths (E). This is 287/246.69 = 1.1634.
5. Multiply the result of O/E by 100. This is 1.1634 × 100 = 116.34 or **116**.

It can therefore be seen that the age-standardised death rate in Mediwell is 116 – that is, 16% higher than that of the standard population of 100.

An SMR should only be compared with the standard population of 100. Therefore SMRs for two or more local populations should not be directly compared with each other.

It is possible to calculate confidence intervals for SMRs. The formula for a 95% confidence interval is as follows:

SMR ± 1.96 × s.e.

$$\text{s.e.} = \left(\frac{\sqrt{O}}{E}\right) \times 100$$

where O = observed and E = expected values. (Source: Bland, 2000)

If the confidence interval does not include 100, we can be 95% confident that the SMR differs significantly from that of the standard population.

Let us calculate confidence intervals for the previous example. We know that the SMR is 116, O = 287 and E = 246.69.

1. Calculate the square root ($\sqrt{}$) of O – this is 16.941.
2. Therefore s.e. = (16.941/246.69) × 100 = 0.069 × 100 = 6.9.
3. 1.96 × s.e. = 1.96 × 6.9 = 13.524.
4. 95% c.i. = 116±13.524 = 116(102.476 → 129.524) or to the nearest whole numbers 116 (102 → 130).

We can see that the confidence interval does not include 100, and we can therefore be 95% confident that the SMR differs significantly from that of the standard population.

A hypothesis test can also be performed to test the null hypothesis that the SMR for the study population = 100 (or in other words, it is the same as that of the standard population, which is always 100). The following formula is used to produce a z-score (*see* Chapter 14):

$z = (O - E)/\sqrt{E}$
(Source: Bland, 2000)

Using the previous example again, we can perform a hypothesis test as follows:

1. Work out the observed value (O) minus the expected (E) = 287 – 246.69 = 40.31.
2. Find the square root of E = $\sqrt{E}$ = $\sqrt{246.69}$ = 15.706.
3. z = 40.31/15.706 = 2.567.
4. Look down each column of the normal distribution table in Appendix 1 to find the z-score (the nearest z-score to 2.567 in the table is 2.57), and then read across to obtain the P-value. The P-value is 0.0102, which is significant.

We can therefore reject the null hypothesis that the SMR for the study population = 100, and use the alternative hypothesis that the SMR is significantly different from that of the standard population.

CHAPTER 26

Measuring association in epidemiology

A number of measures are used to compare the rates of a particular disease experienced by people who have been exposed to a risk factor for that disease and those who have not. For example, if we suspect that smoking is a risk factor for angina, how much more prevalent is angina among those who smoke than among those who do not?

The most widely used measures of association include **absolute risk, relative risk, odds ratio, attributable risk, population attributable risk** and **number needed to treat**.

A **2 × 2 table** can be useful for calculating some measures of association. As we have already seen in Chapter 20, this splits data up into a number of cells, as shown in Table 26.1.

TABLE 26.1 A 2 × 2 table for risk

		Disease present?		
		Yes	No	Total
Exposed to risk factor?	Yes	a	b	a + b
	No	c	d	c + d
	Total	a + c	b + d	a + b + c + d

This 2 × 2 table shows:

- how many patients had a particular disease (cells $a + c$)
- how many did not have the disease ($b + d$)
- how many were exposed to a particular risk factor ($a + b$)
- how many were not exposed to that risk factor ($c + d$)
- how many had the disease, and were exposed to the risk factor (a)

- how many did not have the disease, but were exposed to the risk factor (*b*)
- how many had the disease, but were not exposed to the risk factor (*c*)
- how many did not have the disease, and were not exposed to the risk factor (*d*)
- the total number of subjects (*a* + *b* + *c* + *d*).

ABSOLUTE RISK

This is the probability of having a disease, for those individuals who were exposed to a risk factor. It is calculated as follows:

$$\frac{\text{number of cases of disease in those exposed}}{\text{number of individuals exposed}}$$

When using a 2 × 2 table, absolute risk can be calculated as $a/(a + b)$.

An example is shown in Table 26.2. In the example, if 90 people were exposed to a risk factor, and 20 of them develop a particular disease, their absolute risk is 20/90 = 0.22 or 22%.

TABLE 26.2 A 2 × 2 table example for calculating absolute risk

		Disease present?		
		Yes	**No**	**Total**
Exposed to risk factor?	**Yes**	20 (*a*)	70 (*b*)	90 (*a* + *b*)
	No	16 (*c*)	94 (*d*)	110 (*c* + *d*)
	Total	36 (*a* + *c*)	164 (*b* + *d*)	200 (*a* + *b* + *c* + *d*)

Absolute risk is of limited practical use, because it takes no account of the risk in those individuals who have **not** been exposed to the risk factor.

RELATIVE RISK

Relative risk (or **RR**) indicates the risk of developing a disease in a group of people who were exposed to a risk factor, relative to a group who were not exposed to it.

It is calculated as follows:

$$\text{relative risk} = \frac{\text{disease incidence in exposed group}}{\text{disease incidence in non-exposed group}}$$

- If RR = 1, there is no association between the risk factor and the disease.
- If RR > 1, there is an **increased** risk of developing the disease, if one is exposed to the risk factor (e.g. disease = lung cancer; risk factor = smoking). It suggests that exposure to the risk factor **may cause** the disease.
- If RR < 1, there is a **decreased** risk of developing the disease, if one is exposed to the risk factor (e.g. disease = colon cancer; risk factor = eating fresh fruit and vegetables). It suggests that exposure to the risk factor **may protect against** the disease.

When using a 2 × 2 table like the one in Table 26.1, relative risk can be calculated as

$$\frac{a/a+b}{c/c+d}$$

Let us work out a relative risk from a real study. Are women who are undergoing *in-vitro* fertilisation more likely to suffer a miscarriage in the first trimester if they have bacterial vaginosis? The data are shown in Table 26.3.

$$RR = \frac{a/a+b}{c/c+d} = \frac{22/61}{27/146} = \frac{0.361}{0.185} = 0.361/0.185 = \mathbf{1.95}$$

This study reports that women who are undergoing *in-vitro* fertilisation are nearly twice (1.95 times) as likely to suffer a miscarriage in the first trimester if they have bacterial vaginosis.

RR should not be calculated for case–control studies (Chapter 30); odds ratio should be used instead, and this is discussed later in the chapter.

TABLE 26.3 A 2 × 2 table showing miscarriage in first trimester and bacterial vaginosis status for women undergoing *in-vitro* fertilisation. Adapted from Ralph *et al.* (1999)

		Miscarriage in first trimester (*disease*)		
		Yes	No	Total
Bacterial vaginosis (*risk factor*)	Yes	22 (a)	39 (b)	61 (a + b)
	No	27 (c)	119 (d)	146 (c + d)
	Total	49 (a + c)	158 (b + d)	207 (a + b + c + d)

ATTRIBUTABLE RISK

Attributable risk (or **AR**) is the excess risk of developing a disease in those who have been exposed to a risk factor compared with those who have not.

Attributable risk is especially useful for making decisions for individuals. For example, how much more likely is an individual to develop liver cirrhosis if he or she drinks heavily?

Attributable risk is calculated as follows:

> disease incidence in exposed group – disease incidence in non-exposed group
> **or**, using a 2 × 2 table: $(a/a + b) – (c/c + d)$.

An attributable risk of 0 indicates that there is no excess risk from exposure. In the previous relative risk example (*see* p. 123), the attributable risk of miscarriage in the first trimester to having bacterial vaginosis is calculated as $(22/61) – (27/146) = 0.361 – 0.185 =$ **0.176**. This figure can be multiplied by 1000 to obtain the excess number of first-trimester miscarriages in women with bacterial vaginosis, which can be attributed to having bacterial vaginosis – this is 176 per 1000. Patients experiencing such events should perhaps be offered help in finding coping strategies, in order to minimise the stressful effects involved. Attributable risk should not be calculated for case–control studies (*see* Chapter 30).

POPULATION ATTRIBUTABLE RISK

This assesses how much of a disease **in the population** can be attributed to exposure to a risk factor. It is sometimes abbreviated to **PAR**.

Population attributable risk can be calculated as:

$$\frac{\text{disease incidence in total population} - \text{disease incidence in non-exposed population}}{\text{disease incidence in total population}}$$

It can be useful to public health practitioners in deciding whether to take steps to control the spread of a disease to which the population is exposed. This formula is not suitable for calculating population attributable risk in case–control studies.

ODDS RATIO

In case–control studies (*see* Chapter 30), we retrospectively find people who have already developed a disease and find controls who do not have the disease but who are otherwise similar. Unfortunately, this means that we do not know how many people were exposed to a risk factor for the disease but did not develop it. For this reason, we cannot assume that our sample is representative of the true population. In these circumstances, the **odds ratio** (or **OR**) is used. The odds ratio figure is interpreted in the same way as relative risk.

The odds ratio is calculated as follows:

$$\text{odds ratio} = \frac{\text{odds that subjects } \textit{with} \text{ disease have been exposed to risk factor}}{\text{odds that subjects } \textit{without} \text{ disease have been exposed to risk factor}}$$

Using a 2 × 2 table, the odds ratio can be calculated as:

$$\frac{a/c}{b/d}$$

For example, is there a relationship between adverse life events and breast cancer? The data are shown in Table 26.4.

$$\text{OR} = \frac{\text{odds of subjects with disease being exposed to risk factor}}{\text{odds of subjects without disease being exposed to risk factor}}$$

$$= \frac{a/c}{b/d} = \frac{19/22}{15/63} = \frac{0.864}{0.238} = 0.864/0.238 = \mathbf{3.63}$$

This study reports that women who have experienced greatly threatening life events in the past 5 years are 3.63 times more likely to develop breast cancer than those who have not.

TABLE 26.4 A 2 × 2 table showing breast cancer and greatly threatening life events for women aged 20–70 years undergoing biopsy for a suspicious breast lesion. Adapted from Chen *et al.* (1995)

		Breast cancer (*disease*)		
		Yes	No	Total
At least one greatly threatening life event in the previous 5 years (*risk factor*)	**Yes**	19 *(a)*	15 *(b)*	34 *(a + b)*
	No	22 *(c)*	63 *(d)*	85 *(c + d)*
	Total	41 *(a + c)*	78 *(b + d)*	119 *(a + b + c + d)*

NUMBER NEEDED TO TREAT

If a new treatment seems to be more effective than an existing one, the **number needed to treat** (abbreviated to **NNT**) can indicate how much better that treatment really is. This technique is often used when analysing the results of randomised controlled trials (*see* Chapter 31).

Number needed to treat is a measurement of a **new treatment's** effectiveness, compared with that of an existing treatment. It represents the number of patients who will need to receive the new treatment, in order to produce **one** additional successful cure or other desirable outcome. NNT may also be regarded as a measure of clinical effort expended in order to help patients to avoid poor outcomes, and is concerned with clinical significance rather than statistical significance (Sackett *et al.*, 1997).

Unlike some statistical techniques, there is no 'threshold of significance' with NNT. Judgement needs to be based on factors such as the NNT value and likely benefits, costs or comparisons with other NNT values. If the NNT is small, the new treatment is likely to be worthwhile. If the NNT is large, the new treatment may not be so effective, and careful thought should be given to its implementation. When evaluating expensive treatments, a small NNT may indicate that consideration should be given to adopting the expensive treatment, especially if the disease concerned is relatively rare (however, this is a value judgement – a life saved from a common disease is just as valuable). A NNT figure for a particular intervention can also be usefully compared with the NNT for a different intervention.

When calculating NNT, we also find a figure called the **absolute risk reduction** (**ARR**). This represents the additional percentage of cures obtained by using the new treatment, compared with the existing treatment. In other words, by using the new treatment you are reducing the patient's risk of not being cured by this percentage.

For example, suppose that 624 out of 807 children with meningitis survive when treated with drug A, while 653 out of 691 children survive when a **new drug**, drug B, is used.

The number needed to treat indicates how many patients would need to receive the new drug B in order to prevent **one additional** death (or to produce one additional survivor).

To calculate the number needed to treat, follow these steps.

1. Find the percentage of patients who had the desired outcome in the existing treatment group (*a*).
2. Find the percentage of patients who had the desired outcome in the new treatment group (*b*).
3. Subtract *b* from *a* to obtain the absolute risk reduction – **note**: only the **difference** between *b* and *a* is needed here, so there is no need to use minus numbers.
4. Divide 100 by this figure, to obtain the number needed to treat.

In the example:

> desired outcome = survival
> existing treatment group (*a*) = drug A
> new treatment group (*b*) = drug B.

1. Percentage of patients who survived on drug A = $624/807 \times 100 = 77.3\%$.
2. Percentage of patients who survived on drug B = $653/691 \times 100 = 94.5\%$.

3. $b - a = 17.2$. This shows that the absolute risk reduction is 17.2%.
4. $100/17.2 = \mathbf{5.8}$. This is usually rounded up to the nearest whole number (i.e. **6**).

This shows that six children with meningitis would need to receive the new drug B in order to prevent one additional death. Because the number needed to treat is small, this may well be worth doing (though other factors such as cost and side effects would also need to be taken into consideration when making such a decision). The absolute risk reduction is 17.2%, showing that patients on drug B are 17.2% less likely to die than if they took drug A.

Although NNT is often used for positive outcomes, it can also be used to describe negative outcomes – in this case it is called number needed to **harm** (NNH). The calculation of NNH is the same as NNT, but the emphasis is on how many patients would need to receive a particular intervention in order to produce one **negative** outcome.

CAUSALITY

Finding an association between the presence of disease and a certain risk factor does not necessarily mean that exposure to the risk factor has caused the disease. Other possible factors and potential causes should be identified and eliminated, including chance findings, biases and confounders. Cohort and case–control studies (*see* Chapters 29 and 30) are normally used to investigate causality, but cannot necessarily prove its existence.

If causality is suspected, the following questions can help to determine the strength of evidence.

1. **Dose–response** – is there an association between the incidence of disease and the amount of exposure to the risk factor?
2. **Strength** – are subjects who have been exposed to the risk factor much more likely to develop the disease than unexposed subjects?
3. **Disease specificity** – does the risk factor apply only to the disease being studied?
4. **Time relationship** – did exposure to the risk factor occur before the disease developed?
5. **Biological plausibility** – is what we know about the relationship between the risk factor and disease consistent with what is already known about their biology?
6. **Consistency** – have other investigators working with other populations at other times observed similar results?
7. **Experimental evidence** – do randomised controlled trials show that an intervention can 'cause' outcomes such as increased survival or decreased disease?

These questions are based on the Bradford-Hill criteria (Bradford-Hill, 1965).

CHAPTER 27

Prevalence studies

Prevalence studies are conducted in order to examine the prevalence of a particular condition at a certain point in time. Also referred to as **cross-sectional studies**, they frequently take the form of **surveys**.

They are often conducted at local level, and are useful for investigating disease trends over time, as well as for health service planning. Although prevalence studies are sometimes used to investigate causality, other study designs such as cohort and case–control studies (discussed in Chapters 29 and 30, respectively) are generally more suitable. Prevalence studies are not very useful for examining diseases which have a short duration. They are comparatively quick and easy to carry out, and are useful for situations where no suitable routinely collected data are available.

As an example, a district may be interested in finding out how many people with coronary heart disease (CHD) reside there. A prevalence study could therefore be commissioned to ascertain the prevalence of CHD. Questions could be asked about the presence of diagnosed CHD, plus areas such as diet, smoking, quality of life, family history of CHD, stroke or diabetes, satisfaction with medical services and opinions about future services. The results could be used to plan future CHD services in the district, allowing health professionals to consider whether current services are appropriate and sufficient. A further prevalence study could be carried out at a later date to investigate whether the prevalence of CHD in the district is changing. A survey to establish levels of depression among students could be used to determine whether additional counselling services and other forms of student support might be useful. A study designed to establish the prevalence of taking regular exercise could be used as part of the planning for a local health promotion programme.

Methods for identifying subjects require careful consideration. Electoral rolls or health authority records are often used for this purpose. Potential biases should be identified and steps taken to minimise their effect. Be aware that individuals may choose not to respond, and there may be systematic differences between the kind of people who respond, and those who do not.

The method of sampling therefore needs to be well planned, and all groups who may have the condition being studied should be included. While non-random sampling can be used, randomised sampling is preferable, as this is more likely to be representative of the population as a whole. Sampling techniques are discussed in Chapters 2 and 3.

The actual questionnaire or data collection instrument and the way in which it will be administered should also be carefully chosen and worded. This is discussed in the next chapter.

SOME ADVANTAGES AND DISADVANTAGES OF PREVALENCE STUDIES

Advantages	Disadvantages
Comparatively cheap and quick.	Not useful for conditions which have a short duration.
Fairly simple to carry out and analyse.	Not the first choice for investigating causality.
Useful for healthcare planning and investigating trends over time.	Sampling and data collection need great care.
Useful when routine data are not available.	

CHAPTER 28

Questionnaires

This is a subject which is often considered to be simple, but in practice questionnaires can be difficult to do well. Furthermore, a badly designed questionnaire can completely undermine the results of a study. It is vitally important to consider what information should be collected and how it can best be obtained. While this chapter is not intended as a complete guide to questionnaire design, the following points should be borne in mind.

PLANNING

Plan everything very carefully. Make sure that everyone involved knows exactly what they should be doing. Think carefully about what information you need to collect, and then consider how this can best be achieved. Make a draft of the tables and reports you would like to produce, and if necessary work backwards towards the data you need to collect. Decide how the questionnaire will be administered – for example, will you send it through the post, ask people to fill it in on your premises or use telephone or face-to-face interviews? Also consider what ethical issues need to be taken into account.

CONTENT

Make sure that the data collected can be analysed. For example, do not ask for dates of birth when you really want to know age (many computer databases can convert dates of birth to ages, but if you will be analysing the data manually, by collecting dates you will waste precious time converting to ages manually). Do not collect unnecessary data, but avoid collecting so little data that useful conclusions cannot be drawn. Try to strike a suitable balance.

On the subject of age, people may consider it more acceptable to tell you which age group they belong to, rather than their actual age. Remember, however, that ages can be converted into age groups, but if you only have age groups to start with, these cannot be converted into actual age values. This is something to consider carefully.

Produce questionnaires and data collection forms in a clear and methodical way. Consider how the data will be analysed. You may wish to use 'yes/no' answers, Likert scales and answer selections in preference to open questions, which can be time-consuming and difficult to analyse.

Remember to keep questionnaires as short as possible. People tend to discard questionnaires that are too long or which look too complicated. Aim for no more than one or two sides of A4 paper if possible.

A better response will usually be obtained if you include a paragraph explaining why the survey is being conducted, and how the information will be used.

Use clear, simple wording, but try to avoid sounding patronising. Minimise the possibility of questions being misunderstood (e.g. the question of 'Are you male or female?' may generate 'yes' answers).

Avoid leading questions (e.g. 'Do you agree that our clinic provides an excellent service?'), or the results will be inaccurate and credibility will be compromised.

Start by asking a simple question that is designed to capture the interest of the respondent. For example, **avoid** beginning with a question such as 'What do you think the hospital's priorities for the next year should be?'. People often react well to the fact that you are taking an interest in them, so it is usually advisable to begin by asking about areas such as their age, sex and occupation. Having said this, it is important to be careful not to put people off by asking too many personal questions at the start.

Designing a good questionnaire is very difficult and time-consuming. It is often better to search for an existing questionnaire/data collection instrument/health measurement scale that has already been tried, tested and validated (in this context, 'validated' means shown capable of accurately measuring what it is required to measure).

Various texts (e.g. Bowling, 2001) and the internet can be used to identify many such 'ready-made' instruments. If appropriate to your proposed study, these can save a great deal of time and effort.

Note that it may be necessary to secure permission to use these, and authors should always be properly acknowledged in your publications and reports.

PILOTING

Carry out a short 'dry run' before sending out the first real questionnaire. Ask a number of friends and colleagues to fill it in first. Even if the questionnaire is inappropriate for them, the results may well reveal bugs and other design problems. Try analysing the data from the pilot, too. It is much easier to make changes at this stage. Starting with a pilot can save you a great deal of pain later – ignore this advice at your peril!

DISTRIBUTION AND COMPLETION

Consider this topic carefully, because the choice of method could crucially affect the level of response.

Postal questionnaires allow subjects plenty of time to complete the forms, in the comfort of their own home. However, it should be remembered that postal questionnaires may achieve a response rate of 25% or less. They are also expensive, because you need to cover the cost of postage to the patient, plus the cost of a stamped addressed envelope. If the questionnaires are numbered, personalised or contain a patient ID, you will be able to work out who has failed to respond, and thus have an opportunity to send a reminder. This not only presents problems of extra cost, but can also potentially compromise confidentiality.

If patients are asked to complete and hand in the form before they leave your premises, a much better response rate can be achieved. Choose this option if possible, and consider making someone available to help patients to fill in the form. Make sure that you have a supply of pens available, too. Interviews can be time-consuming and expensive, especially if the interviewer has to visit the subject's home. Telephone interviews are more impersonal, but are less costly in terms of time and money.

When using interviewers, ensure that they all receive training in how to administer the questionnaire. For example, they should be aware that each question should be delivered in the same way by each interviewer. Furthermore, interviewers should not ask leading questions or attempt to interpret answers for respondents. Failure to administer the questionnaire correctly will result in bias (*see* Chapter 24).

QUESTIONS

A range of different types of question are available, including the following.

Fill-in answer

Example: How old are you? _____ years

Yes/No

Example: Do you feel that the physiotherapist has spent long enough with you? (Tick **one** box)

☐ Yes   ☐ No

Selection of answers

Example: How long did you have to wait in the clinic before you were seen by the physiotherapist? (Tick **one** box)

☐ Less than 10 minutes
☐ Between 10 minutes and half an hour

☐ Over half an hour

Likert scales

This is a method of answering a question by selecting one of a range of numbers or responses (e.g. 1 = excellent, 2 = good, 3 = fair, 4 = bad, 5 = very bad) in preference to open questions which can yield large amounts of text that is time-consuming and difficult to analyse.

Example: How do you rate the overall service you received at the physiotherapy clinic? (Tick **one** box)

☐ Excellent   ☐ Good   ☐ Fair   ☐ Bad   ☐ Very bad

Likert scales can have either an even or an odd number of responses. Using an odd number gives respondents the chance to opt for the middle ground (e.g. a choice of excellent/good/fair/bad/very bad allows them to say that they are neither happy nor unhappy, by choosing 'fair'). Using an even number avoids this option, compelling them to go either one way or the other. You need to decide which approach is best for a particular situation.

Open questions

These can provide much more detailed and precise information than other types of question, but they are difficult to analyse. Asking 70 people to tell you about problems they encountered with the service from your department will probably result in most responses being worded differently. Furthermore, some responders may make several separate points in the same answer. You can, of course, group the responses into categories (e.g. 'receptionist was rude – 3', 'no toilet facilities – 5', 'long waiting times – 10', etc.), but you then risk misinterpreting some responses, which can result in bias.

Example: If you encountered any problems with our service, please state them below:

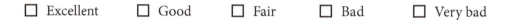

. . . .

. . . .

. . . .

CONFIDENTIALITY

It is good practice to emphasise confidentiality. Reassure patients that their future medical care will not be affected by their response. If you need to incorporate a patient name or ID on the form, explain that this is being done to aid the administration of possible reminders, and that it will not affect confidentiality.

Finally, remember that questionnaires (particularly those dealing with patient satisfaction) are sometimes regarded as 'happy-sheets'. Respondents tend to err on the side of 'happiness', possibly because they do not want to upset anyone or they are concerned about receiving poor treatment in the future. Phrase your questionnaire with this in mind (e.g. by adding a section that stresses confidentiality and/or anonymity), in order to maximise your chances of securing accurate and honest answers).

CHAPTER 29

Cohort studies

Whereas prevalence studies aim to describe how much disease is present at a particular point in time, cohort and case–control studies aim to explore what may have **caused** the disease in the first place.

The first type of study to investigate disease causality is the cohort study (also called the **longitudinal** or **prospective** study). A number of subjects (the **study cohort**) are divided into two groups, namely those who have been exposed to a risk factor and those who have not. The risk factor will be an exposure which is suspected of causing a particular disease. At the beginning of the study, members of the study cohort have similar characteristics and do not appear to have the disease.

A cohort study is usually conducted prospectively (**looking forward in time**), and over a long period. Subjects in the study cohort are followed up over a period of time. The information that is collected on exposure to the risk factor can then be analysed in order to ascertain how many subjects, both exposed and not exposed, develop the disease. If there is an excess of disease in the exposed group, it might be possible to draw conclusions as to whether exposure to the risk factor is causal.

Figure 29.1 shows how a prospective cohort study works.

Suppose that you want to conduct a cohort study to evaluate whether drinking more than five cups of coffee per day in pregnancy leads to fetal abnormalities. First, the local hospital (or better still, a number of hospitals) could provide a list of all newly pregnant women who could be invited to participate in the study. Information could be sought on many factors, including smoking, alcohol consumption, various dietary aspects, exercise, family history of fetal abnormalities, ethnic group and, of course, the number of cups of coffee consumed per day. Some of this information could be used to control for confounding. The women would then be followed up, in order to determine how many give birth to babies with fetal abnormalities. If a high number of mothers with abnormal babies had drunk more than five cups of coffee per day (and there were no significant trends in other factors under observation which might explain the abnormalities), then it might be possible that there is an association between excess coffee drinking and fetal abnormalities.

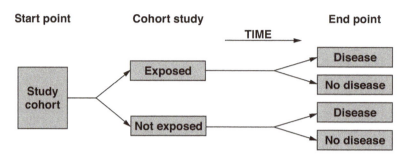

FIGURE 29.1 Prospective cohort study. After Donaldson and Donaldson (2000).

RETROSPECTIVE COHORT STUDIES

Retrospective cohort studies are also possible, and are common in occupational epidemiology and disease outbreak investigations. These, in effect, are prospective cohort studies **in reverse**, as depicted in Figure 29.2. Start points, exposure groups and end points are all treated in the same way – the real difference is that retrospective cohort studies **look back in time**, rather than forward.

For example, we may wish to study whether there is a difference in the quality of care that Asian patients with diabetes have received, relative to non-Asians. It may be that the study needs to be completed quickly, and/or that local GP practices are willing to share their **existing** records containing the data of interest. For this study, exposure is being either Asian or non-Asian. The outcome is whether subjects have received good quality of care (yes/no). GP records will be retrospectively examined (looking back in time), and a judgement on outcome could be made based on whether a number of recommended diabetes checks (such as checks on feet, eyes, $HbA1_c$, etc.) have been done. If a larger proportion of Asians receive the checks (relative to non-Asians), it might be possible to conclude that Asians receive a better standard of care.

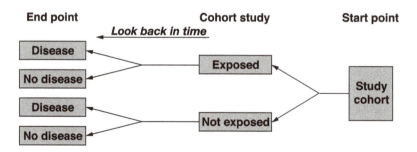

FIGURE 29.2 Retrospective cohort study.

Of course, great care needs to be taken in the design of the study, sample selection and analysis of data. It is vital to look out for possible sources of bias and confounding, and to allow for these.

SUBJECTS

Always think carefully about the aims of the study, and what types of subjects should be chosen. Members of the study cohort should be similar, apart from their exposure to the risk factor. Subjects must not have the disease of interest at the start of the study, and it is important that no population groups are systematically missed. In the previous example, the study cohort is made up of pregnant women. Other studies might use cohorts composed of workers in a certain industry, people in a specific age group or residents in a particular location.

DATA COLLECTION

In the study design, thought should be given to the right method of data collection. Would a questionnaire suffice, or should interviews involving specially trained staff be conducted? Will clinical investigations be necessary? Data should be collected on other factors or characteristics which might have a bearing on the outcome. It is vital to be as clear as possible about what these are, before the study begins, as it may be impossible to collect them at a later stage. The same items of data should be collected for both groups, so that like-for-like comparisons can be made.

FOLLOW-UP

Because cohort studies are usually conducted over a period of time (sometimes several years), they are prone to follow-up bias. The follow-up stage of the study therefore requires careful planning. An agreement needs to be reached on how often follow-up should take place. It may be necessary to follow up at regular intervals, or only at the end of the study. If the disease of interest has a long latent period, a long follow-up period will be needed. Subjects may move away, die or be lost in other ways. Investigators, too, may move on to other jobs, so that continuity is lost. A strategy for tracing subjects should therefore be carefully drawn up, and a plan agreed for investigators to effectively 'hand over' all details of data, methodologies and other information if they leave the study.

DATA ANALYSIS

Relative risk should be used in a cohort study to assess the likelihood of developing the disease in subjects who have been exposed to the risk factor, relative to those who have not been exposed to it. Attributable and population attributable risks can also be calculated, and the Chi-squared test can be employed. However, care needs to be taken when interpreting results, as a strong association does not necessarily indicate a causal relationship. The criteria for causality described in Chapter 26 should also be used.

SOME ADVANTAGES AND DISADVANTAGES OF COHORT STUDIES

Advantages	Disadvantages
Allow outcomes to be explored over time.	Can take a very long time to complete.
The incidence of disease in both exposed and non-exposed groups can be measured.	Diseases with long latent periods may need many years of follow-up.
Useful for rare exposures.	Not so useful for rare diseases.
Can examine the effects of more than one exposure.	Can be very expensive.
More representative of the true population than case–control studies (*see* Chapter 30).	Careful follow-up of all subjects is vital.

Case–control studies

The aim of a case–control study is to assess whether **historical** exposure to one or more risk factors in people who **have** a disease is comparable to that in people who **do not have** the disease. By making this comparison, it may be possible to establish whether exposure to the particular risk factor was associated with the disease in question, and to examine any inter-relationships.

Case–control studies are generally easier and quicker to complete than cohort studies. However, they are prone to certain biases. Whereas cohort studies are usually **prospective (looking forward in time)**, case–control studies are **retrospective (looking back in time)**.

In a case–control study, a number of cases are assembled, consisting of subjects who already have a known disease. In addition, a number of **controls** are gathered who do not have the disease, but who are similar in other respects. Both groups are then investigated in order to ascertain whether they were exposed to a particular risk factor. If an excess of the 'cases' have been exposed to the risk factor, then it **might** be possible that exposure to the risk factor caused the disease.

Figure 30.1 shows how a case–control study works.

For example, suppose that you wish to investigate whether eating fresh fruit and vegetables protects against colorectal cancer. This study is a little different to other examples, as it investigates a protective effect rather than a causal one. Nevertheless, the basic principles are the same. First, a number of patients who had developed colorectal cancer would be selected, as well as a group of subjects who did not have colorectal cancer, but who were similar in other respects. Both groups would be investigated in order to determine whether their diets had included regular amounts of fresh fruit and vegetables, and for how long. If an association was found between cases and controls in the proportion who ate fruit and vegetables regularly, it might be possible to establish that regular consumption of fresh fruit and vegetables has a protective effect against colorectal cancer.

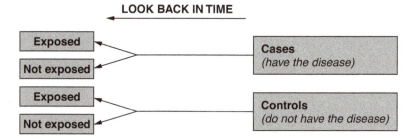

FIGURE 30.1 Case–control study. After Donaldson and Donaldson (2000).

SUBJECTS

Two types of subjects need to be identified, namely cases and controls. At the outset, it is useful to agree explicit criteria on what type of patients should be regarded as cases. For example, in a study of patients with diabetes, it would be important to decide whether 'cases' are patients with insulin-dependent diabetes mellitus (IDDM, or type 1 diabetes) or non-insulin-dependent diabetes mellitus (NIDDM, or type 2 diabetes), or both. It also needs to be decided whether cases should be selected from the population as a whole, or from certain groups (e.g. based on ethnicity, age or sex). The next stage is to determine how these cases can be identified. It is best to use newly diagnosed (**incident**) cases if possible.

Controls should be similar to the cases in every respect other than actually having the disease. Selection bias can occur if there are systematic differences in the way in which cases and controls are recruited into the study. If the study is being conducted on hospital patients, then hospital-based patients without the disease should be selected as controls. If cases are population based, then population-based controls should be used. It can be easier and cheaper to use hospital patients, as a better response can be achieved, and recall bias is minimised. However, problems may be encountered with different exposures being experienced in different hospitals. Furthermore, patients in hospital are ill, and so may not represent the population as a whole. It may sometimes be desirable to use more than one control group if there is uncertainty about the relationship between disease and exposure.

If large differences exist with regard to the age or sex structure of the cases and controls, this could seriously affect the accuracy of any comparisons that are made between them. In order to make the groups more comparable and help to reduce confounding, it is often desirable to **match** each case to one or more controls. It is usual to match cases to controls with regard to age, sex and possibly other factors, according to the design of the study. However, it is unwise to match on too many factors, as this may artificially alter the characteristics of the subjects who are selected.

DATA COLLECTION

In a case–control study, data are collected by surveying subjects (usually by interview) or collecting information from medical records.

Recall bias is a particular problem in case–control studies. For example, patients who have a disease are more likely to recall exposures than patients who have not. Interviews should be structured, asking exactly the same questions of all patients. However, the fact that data are collected retrospectively means that there is likely to be a certain amount of inaccuracy in the information provided by both groups.

When examining medical records, it is important to remember that data on certain risk factors may be more likely to have been recorded in cases than in controls (e.g. alcohol consumption in patients with liver cirrhosis).

If any cases have died or cannot be interviewed for some other reason, it may be possible to collect data from their friends or relatives. Potential biases should be identified and taken into account.

DATA ANALYSIS

The odds ratio should normally be used in a case–control study. The Chi-squared test can also be employed. However, care needs to be taken when interpreting results, as a strong association does not necessarily indicate a causal relationship. The criteria for causality described in Chapter 26 should also be used.

SOME ADVANTAGES AND DISADVANTAGES OF CASE–CONTROL STUDIES

Advantages	**Disadvantages**
Quicker and cheaper to conduct than cohort studies.	Data are retrospective and therefore prone to both selection and information biases.
Allow investigation of more than one risk factor.	Difficult to establish the time between exposure and development of disease.
Especially suitable for rare diseases.	Subjects do not usually represent the population as a whole, so incidence rates cannot be calculated.
Useful for diseases with long latent periods.	Cannot examine the relationship between one possible cause and several diseases.

CHAPTER 31

Randomised controlled trials

Whereas cohort and case–control studies aim to establish what has caused a disease, **randomised controlled trials** (also called **RCTs**) are conducted in order to examine the effectiveness of a particular **intervention**. These are also referred to as **comparative** or **experimental studies** or **clinical trials**. Groups of subjects are recruited by being randomly selected to receive a particular intervention or treatment. RCTs are usually conducted in order to compare the effectiveness of a specific treatment against one or more others. They may also be used for **preventional** (or prophylactic) interventions.

For example, imagine that you wish to compare the effectiveness of a new anticancer drug with a current treatment. A group of patients would be randomly assigned to receive the new drug (group A), and the remainder would be given an existing drug (group B). Detailed records would be maintained on factors such as length of survival, side effects experienced and quality of life. At the end of the trial, the results for group A would be compared with those for group B, and conclusions would be drawn as to which drug was most effective.

Usually two groups of subjects are studied – those who receive the treatment of interest and those who do not. However, some trials use three or more groups. Very often, a new treatment will be compared with an existing one, or even with a **non-treatment** called a **placebo**. A **placebo** is effectively a dummy treatment which appears to be real. Some RCTs are said to be **blind**. This means that the patients do not know whether they have been allocated to the group receiving a new treatment, or an old one, or a placebo. A **double-blind** RCT is one in which neither the patients nor the medical staff know which intervention has been allocated. The practice of blinding reduces the likelihood of patients' outcomes being influenced by their expectation that a new treatment is better or worse, and excludes the possibility of medical staff managing patients differently if they know that a certain therapy is being given, whether or not they actually realise it.

In some trials, subjects may receive one intervention for a certain period, and then be changed over to another intervention. This can be useful when treatment is subjective rather than curative (e.g. for short-term symptom relief), and is known as a **cross-over trial**. It may also be desirable to match pairs of patients on certain characteristics (e.g. age, sex, tumour staging, disease on left- or right-hand side).

Multi-centre trials involve studying subjects at more than one site. They will increase the sample size, and are especially useful when insufficient numbers of subjects can be found at a single site to meet the calculated sample size required.

Unless it is very large, it is unlikely that a single RCT will be able to demonstrate efficacy adequately. The evidence will be stronger if more than one RCT obtains similar results.

STUDY DESIGN

Before commencing an RCT, it is important to agree the explicit **eligibility criteria** for deciding what types of subjects are to be included (based on the characteristics of the disease and the subjects to be studied). If only those patients who are most likely to benefit from the treatment are selected, it should be remembered that they will not represent the whole population of patients with that particular disease. A decision should also be made as to what will constitute the end of the trial (e.g. changes in subjects' condition, death or other physical status). A strict and detailed protocol should be drawn up which describes the exact features of the trial, the outcomes to be recorded, the treatments and controls to be used, how these will be used and what records will be kept. Once the trial starts, subjects in both treatment and control groups are followed up until the end-point is reached. It is likely that an RCT will need a large sample of subjects. The actual sample size required should be calculated. This may be done using formulae which are not included in this basic text, although the basic elements of sample size calculation are discussed in Chapter 21.

Ethical issues should be carefully considered at the planning stage. Subjects should not be exposed to known or potential hazards. It may be unacceptable to withhold treatment from subjects in a control group (e.g. it is obviously unethical not to treat patients who have been diagnosed with cancer). Codes of practice such as those set out in the *Declaration of Helsinki* (World Medical Association, 2013) and others published by various organisations provide guidelines for dealing with ethical issues. It will almost certainly be necessary to seek approval from one or more local research ethics committees before commencing a trial. Potential subjects should always be told about the wish to enter them into the trial, and given full details on how the trial will be conducted. They should be informed and their written consent obtained **before** they are randomised into treatment groups.

If one treatment proves to be significantly superior before the agreed end-point is reached, the trial is sometimes stopped, although the decision as to whether to stop is complex and is best taken by experts.

SUBJECTS

The sample of subjects should be representative of the population as a whole.

Before entering the trial, subjects are **randomly allocated** to a particular **treatment arm**. This aims to ensure that their personal characteristics have no influence over the treatment arm to which they are allocated. Random number tables are often used to allocate patients to treatment groups. For example, the first number in the table can be allocated to the first patient, the second number to the second patient, and so on. Odd numbers may be allocated to treatment group A, and even numbers to treatment group B. The outcomes of patients who are given a particular treatment are compared with those of patients in one or more **control** groups.

If small numbers of patients are involved, or if there are many prognostic factors affecting how individual patients will respond (e.g. age, sex, ethnicity), it may be desirable to use **stratified allocation**. This method involves randomising separately for each prognostic factor. A technique called **block randomisation** (also known as **restricted randomisation**) can be used to ensure that there are equal numbers of subjects in each treatment arm throughout all stages of recruitment. This is achieved by randomising subjects in small blocks. For example, randomisation could be carried out in blocks of six subjects at a time, where three subjects receive treatment A and three receive treatment B.

Randomisation is essential, as it aims to remove bias introduced by patients' individual characteristics. This makes it more likely that only the effect of the treatment will influence the results. The process also helps to reduce **allocation bias** in the selection of subjects (e.g. preventing a clinician from selecting only healthier patients to receive a new treatment). Randomisation controls for known and, more importantly, unknown confounders if the sample size is large enough.

Once subjects have been allocated to a particular group, they should be analysed as part of that group – regardless of whether they comply with their treatment or leave the trial. This is known as being analysed on an **intention-to-treat** basis. This means that data are analysed according to how the subjects were originally intended to be treated. If subjects who refuse to accept the experimental treatment are given (and analysed on) an alternative treatment, this results in bias and will reduce the power of the trial's results.

DATA COLLECTION

Data need to be collected at agreed points throughout the trial. It is advisable to check patient compliance with any treatments given, including placebos. Information will be needed about many factors, including any side effects of treatment.

DATA ANALYSIS AND REPORTING

For continuous data: hypothesis tests, confidence intervals.

For categorical data: Chi-squared test, relative risk, odds ratio, number needed to treat.

For other outcome variables (e.g. trials of independent groups, paired or matched studies, cross-over trials), different methods exist which are not described in this basic guide.

The CONsolidated Standards of Reporting Trials (CONSORT) 2010 Statement is a set of evidence-based recommendations for reporting RCTs, and incorporates a useful checklist (CONSORT, 2010).

SOME ADVANTAGES AND DISADVANTAGES OF RANDOMISED CONTROLLED TRIALS

Advantages	Disadvantages
Allow effectiveness of a new treatment to be evaluated.	Expensive and complicated to perform.
Provides strong evidence of effectiveness.	Patients may refuse treatment – non-compliance can affect results.
Less prone to confounding than other study designs.	A large sample size is needed.
	Careful attention to ethical issues is needed.
	Informed patient consent is essential.

CHAPTER 32

Screening

Screening is performed in order to identify whether people have a disease for which they currently have no symptoms. Screening is not carried out to diagnose illness. Instead, it aims to improve the outcomes of those who are affected, by detecting a disease before its symptoms have developed. If the disease can be diagnosed and treated at an early stage, illness and mortality can be reduced.

A screening test should be able to detect disease in the period between the time when it can be detected using a screening test and the time when symptoms develop.

In practice, screening tests are never completely accurate. There will always be a number of **false-positive** results (in which the test indicates that a subject has the disease when in reality they do not). **False-negative** results can also occur (in which the test indicates that there is no disease present, when in reality the subject **does** have the disease). A good screening test should keep false-positive and false-negative results to an absolute minimum.

Since 1996, all new screening programmes have had to be reviewed by the UK National Screening Committee before they can be introduced in the UK and then continue to be reviewed on a regular basis. Every screening programme is reviewed against a set of 22 criteria (*see* following), including the disease, the test, treatment options and effectiveness, and the acceptability of the screening programme. The criteria are based on those first formulated by the World Health Organization (Wilson and Jungner, 1968), but have been updated to take into account current evidence-based standards and concerns about adverse effects. The findings of up-to-date research are used to ensure that the proposed screening test is both effective **and** cost-effective. Expert groups and patient representatives also form part of the process.

Nevertheless, many people have unrealistically high expectations of screening programmes. There is often a dangerous misconception that a negative test result guarantees that no disease is present. Moreover, if a screening programme does not fulfil all of the criteria, it could do more harm than good (e.g. if patients were expected to undergo a test which had a risk of serious side effects, or if the test is unreliable).

THE UK NATIONAL SCREENING COMMITTEE'S CRITERIA FOR APPRAISING THE VIABILITY, EFFECTIVENESS AND APPROPRIATENESS OF A SCREENING PROGRAMME (REPRODUCED WITH PERMISSION)

Ideally, all of the following criteria should be met before screening for a condition is initiated.

1. The condition

1.1 The condition should be an important health problem.

1.2 The epidemiology and natural history of the condition, including development from latent to declared disease, should be adequately understood and there should be a detectable risk factor, disease marker, latent period or early symptomatic stage.

1.3 All of the cost-effective primary prevention interventions should have been implemented as far as practicable.

1.4 If the carriers of a mutation are identified as a result of screening the natural history of people with this status should be understood, including the psychological implications.

2. The test

2.1 There should be a simple, safe, precise and validated screening test.

2.2 The distribution of test values in the target population should be known and a suitable cut-off level defined and agreed.

2.3 The test should be acceptable to the population.

2.4 There should be an agreed policy on the further diagnostic investigation of individuals with a positive test result and on the choices available to those individuals.

2.5 If the test is for mutations the criteria used to select the subset of mutations to be covered by screening, if all possible mutations are not being tested, should be clearly set out.

3. The treatment

3.1 There should be an effective treatment or intervention for patients identified through early detection, with evidence of early treatment leading to better outcomes than late treatment.

3.2 There should be agreed evidence-based policies covering which individuals should be offered treatment and the appropriate treatment to be offered.

3.3 Clinical management of the condition and patient outcomes should be optimised by all health care providers prior to participation in a screening programme.

4. The screening programme

4.1   There should be evidence from high quality Randomised Controlled Trials that the screening programme is effective in reducing mortality or morbidity. Where screening is aimed solely at providing information to allow the person being screened to make an 'informed choice' (e.g. Down's syndrome, cystic fibrosis carrier screening), there must be evidence from high quality trials that the test accurately measures risk. The information that is provided about the test and its outcome must be of value and readily understood by the individual being screened.

4.2 There should be evidence that the complete screening programme (test, diagnostic procedures, treatment/intervention) is clinically, socially and ethically acceptable both to health professionals and the public.

4.3 The benefit from the screening programme should outweigh the physical and psychological harm (caused by the test, diagnostic procedures and treatment).

4.4 The opportunity cost of the screening programme (including testing, diagnosis and treatment, administration, training and quality assurance) should be economically balanced in relation to expenditure on medical care as a whole (i.e. value for money). Assessment against this criteria should have regard to evidence from cost benefit and/or cost effectiveness analyses and have regard to the effective use of available resource.

4.5 All other options for managing the condition should have been considered (e.g. improving treatment, providing other services), to ensure that no more cost effective intervention could be introduced or current interventions increased within the resources available.

4.6 There should be a plan for managing and monitoring the screening programme and an agreed set of quality assurance standards.

4.7 Adequate staffing and facilities for testing, diagnosis, treatment and programme management should be made available prior to the commencement of the screening programme.

4.8 Evidence-based information explaining the consequences of testing, investigation and treatment should be made available to potential participants to assist them in making an informed choice.

4.9 Public pressure for widening the eligibility criteria, for reducing the screening interval, and for increasing the sensitivity of the testing process, should be anticipated. Decisions about these parameters should be scientifically justifiable to the public.

4.10 If screening is for a mutation the programme should be acceptable to people identified as carriers and to other family members.

National programmes in the UK include screening for breast cancer, bowel cancer, cervical cancer, abdominal aortic aneurysm, chlamydia, plus antenatal and neonatal conditions. There is currently some debate concerning whether programmes should be established for diseases such as prostate cancer. The NHS Health Check Programme is offered to people aged between 40 and 74, aimed at helping to prevent heart disease, stroke, kidney disease, diabetes and dementia. Other screening takes place in various settings, such as eye tests for certain patients with disabilities and tests for diabetes.

EVALUATING THE ACCURACY OF SCREENING TESTS

A screening test can be evaluated using a **2 × 2 table**, as shown in Table 32.1. It shows:

- how many subjects with a positive result actually have the disease (**true positive**) (cell a)
- how many subjects with a positive result do not have the disease (**false positive**) (b)
- how many subjects have a positive result ($a + b$)
- how many subjects have a negative result ($c + d$)
- how many subjects with a negative result actually have the disease (**false negative**) (c)
- how many subjects with a negative result do not have the disease (**true negative**) (d)
- how many subjects actually have the disease ($a + c$)
- how many subjects do not have the disease ($b + d$)
- the total number of subjects ($a + b + c + d$).

TABLE 32.1 A 2 × 2 table for evaluating a screening test

		Disease status		
		Present	Absent	Total
Result of screening test	**Positive**	a True positive	b False positive	$a + b$
	Negative	c False negative	d True negative	$c + d$
	Total	$a + c$	$b + d$	$a + b + c + d$

There are a number of ways to measure the accuracy of a screening test. The most commonly used methods are described following.

Sensitivity

This is the proportion of subjects who really have the disease, and who have been identified as diseased by the test.

The formula for calculating sensitivity is $a/(a + c)$.

Specificity

This is the proportion of subjects who really do not have the disease, and who have been identified as non-diseased by the test.

The formula for calculating specificity is $d/(b + d)$.

Sensitivity and specificity both indicate how accurately the test can detect whether or not a subject has the disease (this is known as the test's **validity**).

Positive predictive value (PPV)

This is the probability that a subject with a positive test result really has the disease.

The formula for calculating PPV is $a/(a + b)$.

Negative predictive value (NPV)

This is the probability that a subject with a negative test result really does not have the disease.

The formula for calculating NPV is $d/(c + d)$.

Prevalence

This is the proportion of diseased subjects in a screened population (also called the **pre-test probability**), and it is the probability of having the disease before the screening test is performed. It can be especially useful when evaluating screening tests for groups of people who may have different prevalences (e.g. different sexes, age groups or ethnic groups).

The formula for calculating prevalence in screening is $(a + c)/(a + b + c + d)$.

Suppose that a new screening test has been developed for diabetic retinopathy. We carry out a study to find out how effective it is in a population of 33 750 patients with diabetes, all aged over 55 years. The results shown in Table 32.2 are produced. Let us use these data to evaluate the test.

TABLE 32.2 A 2 × 2 table for evaluating a diabetic retinopathy screening test

		Diabetic retinopathy		
		Present	Absent	Total
Result of screening test	**Positive**	3200 (a)	1400 (b)	4600 (a + b)
	Negative	150 (c)	29 000 (d)	29 150 (c + d)
	Total	3350 (a + c)	30 400 (b + d)	33 750 (a + b + c + d)

- **Sensitivity** = $a/(a + c)$ = 3200/3350 = **0.9552** = 96%.
  This means that 96% of subjects who actually have diabetic retinopathy will be correctly identified by the test. This result indicates that only 4% of subjects with diabetic retinopathy will be wrongly identified as being disease-free.
- **Specificity** = $d/(b + d)$ = 29 000/30 400 = **0.9539** = 95%.
  This means that 95% of subjects who **do not have** diabetic retinopathy will be correctly identified by the test. This result indicates that only 5% of subjects without the disease will be wrongly identified as having diabetic retinopathy.
- **PPV** = $a/(a + b)$ = 3200/4600 = **0.6957** = 70%.
  This means that there is a 70% chance that someone who tests positive does have diabetic retinopathy. This is poor, as there is a 30% chance that someone with a positive test result is actually disease-free.
- **NPV** = $d/(c + d)$ = 29 000/29 150 = **0.9949** = 99%.
  This means that there is a 99% chance that someone who tests negative **does not have** diabetic retinopathy. This is good, as there is only a 1% chance that someone with a negative test result will actually have the disease.
- **Prevalence** = $(a + c)/(a + b + c + d)$ = 3350/33 750 = **0.0993** = 10%.
  This means that 10% of the screened population have diabetic retinopathy.

We can conclude that although this screening test appears to be generally very good, the disappointing PPV of only 70% would limit its overall usefulness.

CHAPTER 33

Evidence-based healthcare

To ensure that patients receive the best healthcare, their clinical management and treatment need to be informed by the current best evidence of effectiveness. This is called **evidence-based healthcare** or EBHC.

EBHC is 'when decisions that affect the care of patients are taken with due weight accorded to all valid, relevant information' (Hicks, 1997). It is closely related to **evidence-based medicine** (EBM), defined by Sackett *et al.* (2000) as 'the integration of best research evidence with clinical expertise and patient values'. Dawes *et al.* (2005) suggested that the concept of EBM should be expanded to **evidence-based practice** (EBP) 'to reflect the benefits of entire health care teams and organisations adopting a shared evidence-based approach'.

The 'Sicily Statement on evidence-based practice' (Dawes *et al.*, 2005) outlines a process of five steps for practicing EBP:

1. translation of uncertainty to an answerable question
2. systematic retrieval of best evidence available
3. critical appraisal of evidence for validity, clinical relevance, and applicability
4. application of results in practice
5. evaluation of performance.

A second Sicily statement, published in 2011, focused on the development of EBP learning assessment tools and proposed the Classification Rubric for EBP Assessment Tools in Education (CREATE) framework for their classification (Tilson *et al.*).

It is therefore important that healthcare professionals develop the skills to follow these steps, which include finding evidence and assessing its quality, before deciding whether it should be applied in practice. The ability to search for literature and critically analyse evidence are essential in order to do this well.

This chapter provides a brief overview of EBHC and associated topics, as well as discussing some of the skills required to use it. Other texts cover this subject in greater detail.

The amount of skill and work required will depend on the situation. For example, a researcher carrying out an in-depth literature review will need to carry out comprehensive or exhaustive searching and analysis. On the other hand, a busy clinician searching for EBHC purposes would be advised to start by searching for existing 'pre-appraised' evidence such as systems, synopses, summaries, systematic reviews, etc. (discussed later in this chapter) that have already summarised and evaluated the primary studies concerned.

LITERATURE SEARCHING

A dazzling array of information sources is available, and can be used to find research papers, reviews of evidence, health economic analyses and other documents. The process of searching can seem very daunting, as there are so many sources of information. A well thought out **search strategy** is therefore vital, and detailed planning is required before actually starting a search. It is important to begin any search with a clear, well-focused and explicit question.

Careful thought should be given as to exactly what to search for, in order to find what is required. For example, if you are looking for evidence on diabetes, are you interested in patients with type 1, type 2 or any type of diabetes? If your research interest is in Asian children with type 1 diabetes, the search may need to be focused on this specific patient group, to avoid finding superfluous information (e.g. middle-aged Caucasians with type 2 diabetes). Also, diabetes is sometimes known as 'diabetes mellitus', so it is worth finding out whether the subject of your search is known by other names, or is spelled differently in other English-speaking countries (for example, 'oesophagus' is spelled 'esophagus', and 'anaemia' is spelled 'anemia' in the USA). Additionally, drugs are sometimes known by different proprietary names (e.g. riluzole's proprietary name is Rilutek®, and the proprietary name of the levonorgestrel-releasing intra-uterine system is Mirena®).

Unfortunately, much valuable information never gets published at all. Investigators sometimes abandon projects before they are completed, or never get around to writing them up and submitting for publication. Some journals may prefer to publish studies that demonstrate positive outcomes – thus overlooking those with negative or neutral results, resulting in a misleading impression of true efficacy. This is a type of bias not previously discussed – **publication bias**. One method of detecting publication bias is to use a **funnel plot** – these plot the treatment effect against a measurement related to the size of the study. If no publication bias is present, the plot should be shaped like a symmetrical inverted funnel, with smaller studies (usually showing a wider spread of treatment effect) at the base and larger studies (usually with less spread) at the neck of the plot. If there is publication bias, the shape of the funnel plot may be skewed and have a characteristic 'hole' in the lower left corner, indicating the absence of small studies with weak or negative treatment effects (Glasziou *et al.*, 2001; Last, 2001; Po, 1998). Also, researchers or organisations funding the research may have hidden the results of studies with negative findings, so that only those with positive results are made public – this is a very unethical and potentially dangerous practice, which can never be condoned. Unpublished evidence can therefore be useful, and should not be ignored out of hand.

'Grey literature' can also be a source of useful information – this includes material such as conference proceedings, newsletters and reports from a range of sources produced by governments, universities, industry and other organisations. Some of the information may be in languages other than English. Although this presents obvious difficulties, it is unwise to assume that that such information will not be useful. Abstracts of foreign papers sometimes appear in English, and colleagues may be able to suggest individuals who can translate. Also, several internet sites offer facilities which can be used to translate blocks of text from various languages into English (such translations are not always completely accurate, however).

In order to find a wide range of evidence on a subject, it may be necessary to search on every possible permutation. Of course, a wider preliminary search may be desirable, so as to find as much information as possible on the whole subject (sometimes called a **scoping search**).

It is necessary to find a balance between spending a substantial amount of time trying to find **every** piece of evidence on a subject and doing less a detailed search in a more manageable timeframe. Comprehensive and exhaustive searching will be needed for researchers conducting a systematic review, though EBHC practitioners looking for evidence on a particular subject are likely to need a more sensitive and efficient search.

For this reason, as previously mentioned, busy clinicians searching for EBHC purposes are advised to start by searching for pre-appraised evidence, such as systems, summaries, synopses or existing systematic reviews, and only look for primary studies (randomised controlled trials (RCTs), cohort studies, etc.) when no systematic reviews are available. This will be discussed further later in this chapter.

The following steps should always be observed.

1. Decide where to search – **electronic databases, appropriate journals, conference proceedings, other sources**.
2. Define some **search terms** to help identify the right literature. Include keywords, alternative names, terms and spellings (e.g. 'diabetes', 'diabetes mellitus', 'Asian', 'adult', 'insulin dependent', 'type 1', 'type I', 'IDDM').
3. Decide on **inclusion and exclusion criteria** – these are an explicit statement of what types of study you will include (e.g. those of patients with pancreatic cancer,

aged 65+), and which you will exclude (e.g. those of children and adults under 65, studies carried out before 1970). It is important to be able to justify the reasons for any inclusions and exclusions – for example, if the search is based on a drug first released in 1982, it may be appropriate to exclude studies published before 1980, though it would be harder to justify excluding non-English literature because researchers could not translate.

4. Seek advice and assistance from medical librarians – they can be a source of considerable expertise and help.

5. Consider identifying and contacting **subject experts** and **authors** of studies in the subject area. They are usually happy to help, and can sometimes provide a wealth of valuable information – especially on unpublished data. This is especially advisable if you are doing a comprehensive and exhaustive search.

Some tips on using electronic databases are presented in Figure 33.1.

The selection of useful electronic literature databases and search engines shown in Figure 33.2 can also be useful. Some are freely available online, while others require

---

- Start with your subject of interest, then convert each element into a series of keywords. Think of synonyms/alternative spellings, e.g. 'neurone'/'neuron'.
- Some databases allow the use of Medical Subject Headings (MeSH) – e.g. 'anaemia – hypochronic'. 'MeSH' is a vocabulary used for indexing articles. MeSH terminology provides a consistent way to retrieve information.
- Find the nearest equivalent indexing terms (MeSH headings – for MEDLINE and Cochrane Library) – look at those in any papers you have already found.
- Use 'AND/OR', e.g. "Asian AND diabetes" shows everyone who is Asian AND has diabetes.
- Search using 'text-words' – words appearing in title or abstract, e.g. iron deficiency anaemia).
- Use a combination of text-words and indexing terms.
- Consider using published predefined search strategies ('filters').
- Compromise between 'sensitivity' (getting everything relevant) and 'specificity' (proportion of hits to hits and misses); to be comprehensive, you must sacrifice specificity.
- If too many records are retrieved – narrow the search:
  — use more specific or the most relevant text-words
  — use MeSH terms rather than text-words
  — select specific sub-headings with MeSH terms.
- If too few records are retrieved, widen the search:
  — use more terms
  — use the 'explosion' feature (if available, this allows you to select a number of broader search terms)
  — select all sub-headings with MeSH terms.

FIGURE 33.1 Tips on using electronic databases for literature searching.

- MEDLINE®: covers the whole field of medical information. Available from several sources (e.g. via Ovid in medical libraries or by corporate subscription) or free at www.ncbi.nlm.nih.gov/pubmed, which also incorporates a 'Clinical Queries' feature that applies filters to specific clinical research areas to achieve greater sensitivity
- The University of York Centre for Reviews and Dissemination: a useful source of information and has three searchable databases – www.york.ac.uk/inst/crd/
- UK Health Technology Assessment Programme: www.ncchta.org/
- UK Clinical Research Network Portfolio: searchable archive of funded NHS research studies – http://public.ukcrn.org.uk/search/
- National Institute for Health and Care Excellence (NICE) Health and Social Care Evidence Search: www.evidence.nhs.uk/
- *Bandolier*: newsletter of literature on healthcare effectiveness – www.medicine.ox.ac.uk/bandolier/
- Department of Health: www.doh.gov.uk
- National Statistics: www.statistics.gov.uk/
- Turning Research Into Practice (Trip) database: www.tripdatabase.com/index.html
- Embase®: for registered users – www.embase.com/
- Science Citation Index: accessible by licensed institutions – http://thomsonreuters.com/science-citation-index-expanded/
- CINAHL Complete: nursing and allied health database, accessible by licensed institutions – www.ebscohost.com/nursing/products/cinahl-databases/cinahl-complete
- Centre for Evidence-Based Medicine (CEBM): www.cebm.net/index.aspx
- The Cochrane Collaboration at the UK Cochrane Centre: www.cochrane.org/. The collaboration aims to improve healthcare decision-making, globally, through systematic reviews, which are published in the Cochrane Library – www.cochranelibrary.com/. The library contains high quality independent evidence to inform healthcare decision-making
- *ACP Journal Club Archives* (free access to issues 1991–2008) www.acpjc.org/
- *The BMJ*: electronic version of all *BMJ* issues since 1994, some of which can be searched free of charge – www.bmj.com/theBMJ
- BMJ *Evidence Based Medicine*: for registered users – http://ebm.bmj.com/
- BMJ *Clinical Evidence*: for registered users – http://clinicalevidence.bmj.com/ceweb/index.jsp
- *The Lancet*: electronic version of *The Lancet* – www.thelancet.com/journals/lancet/issue/current
- Critically appraised topics (or CATs): summaries of evidence for specific clinical questions. An internet search will reveal many of these, some of which are arranged into 'CAT banks'
- Internet search engines, for example:
  - Bing – www.bing.com/
  - Google – www.google.com/
  - Google Scholar – www.google.com/scholar
  - Yahoo – https://uk.yahoo.com/.

FIGURE 33.2 A selection of useful internet sites and databases for literature searching.

a paid subscription so may therefore only be available through subscribing medical libraries, academic institutions and healthcare organisations.

When a search has been carried out, the literature identified should be screened to exclude any texts which do not meet the predefined inclusion criteria. Some papers can be excluded on the basis of their title or abstract, while it may be necessary to obtain full copies of others. It is good practice to note the number of papers identified, the number excluded (including reasons for exclusion) and the number used in the final literature review. A flow diagram, such as that shown in Figure 33.3, can be useful to summarise this information. The Preferred Reporting Items for Systematic Reviews and Meta-Analyses (PRISMA) Statement (Moher *et al.*, 2009, discussed later in this chapter) includes a flow diagram that is also appropriate here.

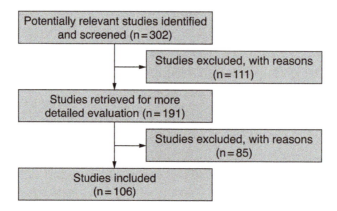

FIGURE 33.3 Flow diagram summarising the number of studies found, excluded and used for a literature review.

The next stage is to critically analyse the papers included to decide whether they contain good quality evidence of effectiveness.

CRITICAL ANALYSIS OF STUDIES

The RCT has traditionally been regarded as the best quality study design to assess effectiveness, but other types can also be useful. The **hierarchy of evidence** lists study types and sources in order, based on the quality of evidence they are likely to provide.

There are many different versions of this hierarchy, which is evolving over time. Figure 33.4 shows that **systematic reviews** and **meta-analyses** are regarded as superior to designs such as RCTs and cohort studies, and that expert opinions, editorials and anecdotes provide the least reliable quality of evidence.

RCTs, cohort, case–control and **prevalence studies** are discussed in earlier chapters. **Case series** are reports based on the observation of a usually small number of

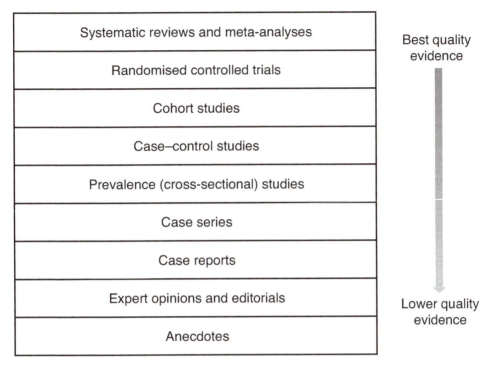

| Systematic reviews and meta-analyses |
| Randomised controlled trials |
| Cohort studies |
| Case–control studies |
| Prevalence (cross-sectional) studies |
| Case series |
| Case reports |
| Expert opinions and editorials |
| Anecdotes |

Best quality evidence

Lower quality evidence

FIGURE 33.4 A hierarchy of evidence.

patients. **Case reports** focus on single patients – a medical journal might publish a case report discussing an unusual presentation of a particular disease in a 17-year-old, for example. Both case series and case reports can be useful for highlighting interesting clinical information, or providing clues as to possible effects of treatment or exposure, but clearly cannot be used to provide robust evidence of effectiveness. **Expert opinion** may be based on long experience, but is not necessarily founded on dependable evidence – indeed, it is sometimes regarded as **eminence-based** (rather than evidence-based) practice. **Editorials** in journals and other publications often present the personal views of the author(s), which may not be evidence based. **Anecdote** typically takes the form of a colleague or friend saying they have been told that eating a certain type of vegetable can prevent cancer, for instance, and clearly cannot in itself be relied upon to provide good quality evidence.

It is important to remember, however, that a well-designed cohort study may actually provide better evidence than a badly conducted RCT, for example. Indeed, the appropriateness of study used, plus quality of study design and execution also needs to be taken into account when assessing the strength of evidence. Another important consideration is that even if well planned and conducted, the strength of evidence from a **single** study is limited by its sample size and generalisability to the population as a whole.

It is increasingly being suggested that other pre-appraised resources can provide even higher quality evidence. The 6S model (DiCenso *et al.*, 2009) has been developed to aid clinical decision-making, and suggests that clinicians seeking evidence should begin by searching for **systems** (computerised decision support systems, linked to individual patient characteristics and current evidence-based guidelines; highest quality evidence). If none is found, they should search for **summaries** (guidelines/ textbooks incorporating the current best evidence from reviews and other studies). In the absence of summaries, **synopses of syntheses** (concise descriptions of several high quality systematic reviews) should be sought. In decreasing order of quality after this come **syntheses** (individual systematic reviews), **synopses of studies** (summaries of a single study, including an appraisal and commentary) and, finally, individual **studies**.

The GRADE (short for Grading of Recommendations Assessment, Development and Evaluation) working group has developed an approach to grade the quality of evidence and the strength of recommendations, and has also published criteria for applying their system (GRADE working group, 2015). Similarly, the PRISMA Statement has been formulated to improve the reporting of systematic reviews and meta-analyses (Moher *et al.*, 2009). The statement includes a useful checklist and flow diagram.

Reliability and **validity** are important factors to be considered when assessing the quality of studies. **Reliability** is the extent to which the results of a measurement or study can be replicated. For a measurement, **validity** refers to how accurately the measurement actually measures what it claims to. The **validity of a study** can be divided into two types – **internal** and **external**. **Internal validity** applies if the differences between study groups are due only to the effect being hypothesised, rather than as a result of confounding or other bias. **External validity** refers to how generalisable the results of a study are to its target population.

Research papers frequently refer to statistical and epidemiological terms such as particular tests and procedures (e.g. 95% confidence interval, P-value, t-tests, χ^2, correlation and linear regression, analysis of variance) and epidemiological terms (e.g. types of epidemiological study, bias, relative risk, odds ratio, number needed to treat, number needed to harm). A good understanding of these terms – **as a minimum** – is therefore essential. Critical appraisal skills contain elements that can be useful for learning how to read and make sense of a paper, how to make judgements about the quality of studies and in planning your own study.

Organisations such as the Critical Appraisal Skills Programme (CASP) have developed templates to assess the quality of a variety of study types including RCTs and systematic reviews, qualitative research, economic reviews, cohort and case–control studies, and diagnostic tests. Their templates all contain questions recommended when critically appraising studies. They are designed as pedagogic tools to be used in discussion groups at CASP workshops, but are available for download on their website. Figure 33.5 shows questions recommended by CASP when assessing reviews.

10 QUESTIONS TO HELP YOU MAKE SENSE OF A REVIEW

How to use this appraisal tool

Three broad issues need to be considered when appraising the report of a systematic review:

- Are the results of the review valid? (Section A)
- What are the results? (Section B)
- Will the results help locally? (Section C)

The 10 questions on the following pages are designed to help you think about these issues systematically.

The first two questions are screening questions and can be answered quickly. If the answer to both is "yes", it is worth proceeding with the remaining questions.

There is some degree of overlap between the questions; you are asked to record a "yes", "no" or "can't tell" to most of the questions. A number of prompts are given after each question. These are designed to remind you why the question is important. Record your reasons for your answers in the spaces provided.

These checklists were designed to be used as educational tools in part of a workshop setting. There will not be time in the small groups to answer them all in detail!

(A) Are the results of the review valid?
Screening Questions

1. Did the review address a clearly focused question?   ☐ Yes   ☐ Can't tell   ☐ No

HINT: An issue can be 'focused' In terms of
- The population studied
- The intervention given
- The outcome considered

2. Did the authors look for the right type of papers?   ☐ Yes   ☐ Can't tell   ☐ No

HINT: 'The best sort of studies' would
- Address the reviews question
- Have an appropriate study design (usually RCTs for papers evaluating interventions)

Is it worth continuing?

Detailed questions

3. Do you think all the important, relevant studies
    were included?   ☐ Yes   ☐ Can't tell   ☐ No

HINT: Look for
- Which bibliographic databases were used
- Follow up from reference lists
- Personal contact with experts
- Search for unpublished as well as published studies
- Search for non-English language studies

4. Did the review's authors do enough to assess
    the quality of the included studies?   ☐ Yes   ☐ Can't tell   ☐ No

HINT: The authors need to consider the rigour of the studies they have identified. Lack of rigour may affect the studies' results. ("All that glisters is not gold" Merchant of Venice – Act II Scene 7)

5. If the results of the review have been combined,
    was it reasonable to do so?   ☐ Yes   ☐ Can't tell   ☐ No

HINT: Consider whether
- The results were similar from study to study
- The results of all the included studies are clearly displayed
- The results of the different studies are similar
- The reasons for any variations in results are discussed

(B) What are the results?

6.   What are the overall results of the review?

HINT: Consider
- If you are clear about the review's 'bottom line' results
- What these are (numerically if appropriate)
- How were the results expressed (NNT, odds ratio etc)

7.   How precise are the results?

HINT: Look at the confidence intervals, if given

(C) Will the results help locally?

8. Can the results be applied to the local population?   ☐ Yes   ☐ Can't tell   ☐ No

HINT: Consider whether
- The patients covered by the review could be sufficiently different to your population to cause concern
- Your local setting is likely to differ much from that of the review

9. Were all important outcomes considered?   ☐ Yes   ☐ Can't tell   ☐ No

HINT: Consider whether
- Is there other information you would like to have seen

10. Are the benefits worth the harms and costs?   ☐ Yes   ☐ Can't tell   ☐ No

HINT: Consider
- Even if this is not addressed by the review, what do you think?

FIGURE 33.5 Questions to be used when assessing the quality of a systematic review – reproduced with permission of the Critical Appraisal Skills Programme (CASP; 2013). © Critical Appraisal Skills Programme (CASP) Systematic Review Checklist, 31 March 2013.

Meta-analysis improves on the quality of evidence, by statistically combining the results of **several** studies. The aim is to extract the data and then 'pool together' the results (providing it is appropriate to do so). As the results of **all** the included trials are taken into account, a better overall picture of evidence can be obtained. The combined results are often summarised using **forest plots** (sometimes also called **blobbograms**). Figure 33.6 shows an example forest plot, summarising the results of a meta-analysis involving four studies.

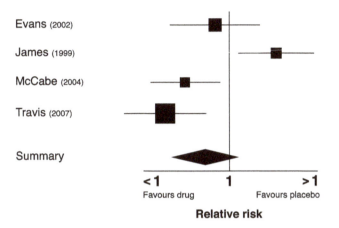

FIGURE 33.6 Example forest plot, showing the results and a summary of four studies.

Going back to Chapter 26, measures of association such as **relative risk** (RR) and **odds ratio** (OR) can be used to compare the experiences of people who have been exposed to a risk factor for a disease, relative to those who have not been exposed. These can also be used in other situations – for example, to measure and compare the effectiveness of treatments. In Figure 33.6, four different studies have evaluated the effectiveness of a particular drug, compared with a placebo. The results of each study are represented by a square or a dot (the RR, in this case) and a line (showing 95% confidence intervals). Larger squares denote larger sample sizes. The **combined** results of this meta-analysis are shown as a diamond shape, where the middle is the RR, with lines showing 95% confidence intervals at either side. As indicated in Figure 33.6, for this study an RR of < 1 means that the drug is more effective than placebo, whereas an RR of > 1 favours the placebo. An RR of exactly 1 means that there is no difference between the two. Going back to the individual studies, it can be seen that those conducted by Travis and McCabe both favour the drug treatment. Furthermore, the confidence intervals for both studies have an RR **below** 1, indicating there is a 95% probability that the population RR is less than 1. The interval does not cross the line of RR = 1. The study by James shows that placebo is more effective – again, both sides of the confidence interval have an RR **above** 1, and do not cross the line. This is important, as if either confidence limit crossed this line, it would mean that the result of the study could favour either the drug **or** the placebo – the results would not therefore be sufficiently accurate to show that either treatment was significantly better than the other. In the Evans study, it can be seen that although the RR favours drug treatment, the confidence intervals cross the RR = 1 line. This is also the case for the overall summary – it can therefore be concluded that there is insufficient evidence that either treatment is more effective than the other. So on the basis of this evidence, neither can be recommended for use in clinical practice.

An important drawback of meta-analyses is that efforts may not have been made to find **every** study on the intervention of interest, resulting in bias (including publication bias). In addition, further important elements, such as the quality of studies, quality of life and cost-effectiveness, may not have been evaluated.

Indeed, effectiveness alone is not enough for a treatment to be adopted into practice. The **clinical effectiveness triangle** shows three elements (efficacy, cost and quality of life), all of which must be acceptable, in order for a treatment to be adopted into routine clinical practice. For example, a treatment that is acceptable in terms of effectiveness and cost is of limited benefit if quality of life is so poor (due to severe side effects) that patients cannot tolerate it. Similarly, a low-cost treatment with few side effects is practically useless if it is not effective.

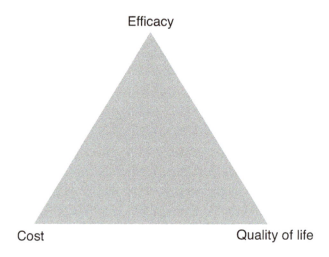

FIGURE 33.7 The clinical effectiveness triangle (Stewart, 2010).

Systematic reviews attempt to overcome the limitations of meta-analysis by systematically seeking out **all** studies – published, unpublished, abandoned and in progress. As well as summarising results (and using graphical methods including forest plots), systematic reviews should evaluate the quality of studies together with quality-of-life and cost-effectiveness data if available. Patient experiences are also sometimes taken into account.

With regard to quality of life, quality-adjusted life years (QALYs) are frequently used in assessing specific healthcare interventions. QALYs combine improvements in the length and quality of life into one single index (Bowling, 1997). Essentially, QALYs estimate the number of remaining years of life following a specific treatment, and apply a weighting for each year with a quality-of-life score between 0 (being dead) and 1 (perfect health) (National Institute for Health and Care Excellence (NICE), 2015; Lewis *et al.*, 2008). The QALY takes 1 year of perfect "health-life expectancy" as being worth a value of 1 (Bowling, 2014). Several criticisms of QALYs have been made, including that they are 'ageist', tending to favour younger people (Harris, 2005; Orme *et al.*, 2003).

Where possible, further analysis and statistical modelling may also be undertaken. In the UK, organisations such as NICE use systematic reviews as part of the process for deciding whether new drugs and health technologies should be used in the NHS.

Both meta-analyses and systematic reviews are also called **overviews**, and are examples of **secondary research** (observational or experimental studies that collect original data from subjects are regarded as **primary research**).

This chapter has not aimed to provide specific guidance on actually carrying out a systematic review or meta-analysis, which is provided by a number of publications – *see* Further reading. The process of undertaking these can be extremely time-consuming and complicated, often requiring specialist skills in several fields (e.g. experts in the condition being studied, systematic review methodology, advanced statistical analysis and health economics). For this reason, they need to be conducted by teams rather than individuals. It is, however, important for healthcare profession-als to understand what systematic reviews are and be able to evaluate their quality.

We have now reached the end of this basic guide to statistics and epidemiology. Hopefully, you will have grasped the main elements of these topics, and you may feel ready to gain a deeper understanding by reading some of the books listed in the Further reading section on page 211. If you work in the field of healthcare, you may even be able to start using your new knowledge in a practical way.

However, before doing this, it might be useful to work through the exercises in Appendix 2. These cover quite a lot of the theories included in this book, and are followed by a full answer guide in Appendix 3.

Glossary of terms

x	A measurement or variable
$\bar{x}$	Sample mean (called 'x-bar')
χ^2	Chi-squared value (from the Chi-squared distribution)
Σ	Add together all of the following values (called 'sigma')
μ	Population mean (called 'mu')
$\sqrt{}$	Square root
σ	Standard deviation for populations
$\pm$	Plus or minus
$/$	Divide by (same as '$\div$')
$\leq$	Less than or equal to
$\geq$	More than or equal to
$<$	Less than
$>$	More than
α	Type 1 error (or 'alpha error')
β	Type 2 error (or 'beta error')
AR	Attributable risk (or absolute risk)
ARR	Absolute risk reduction
CI or c.i.	Confidence interval
d	Cohen's d statistic
d.f.	Degrees of freedom
EBHC	Evidence-based healthcare
EBM	Evidence-based medicine
EBP	Evidence-based practice
N or n	Sample size
NNH	Number needed to harm
NNT	Number needed to treat
NPV	Negative predictive value
OR	Odds ratio
P or p	Probability or significance value
p	Observed proportion
ρ	Spearman's rank correlation coefficient
PAR	Population attributable risk
PPV	Positive predictive value
r	Pearson's product moment correlation coefficient

RCT	Randomised controlled trial
RR	Relative risk
s	Standard deviation for samples
SD or s.d.	Standard deviation
SE or s.e.	Standard error
SMR	Standardised mortality ratio
t	t-value (from the t-distribution)
τ	Tau, as in Kendall's τ
z	Test statistic used in the normal test

Statistical tables

NORMAL DISTRIBUTION: TWO-TAILED AREAS (ALTMAN, 1991)
REPRODUCED WITH PERMISSION

z	P	z	P	z	P	z	P
0.00	1.0000						
0.01	0.9920	0.31	0.7566	0.61	0.5419	0.91	0.3628
0.02	0.9840	0.32	0.7490	0.62	0.5353	0.92	0.3576
0.03	0.9761	0.33	0.7414	0.63	0.5287	0.93	0.3524
0.04	0.9681	0.34	0.7339	0.64	0.5222	0.94	0.3472
0.05	0.9601	0.35	0.7263	0.65	0.5157	0.95	0.3421
0.06	0.9522	0.36	0.7188	0.66	0.5093	0.96	0.3371
0.07	0.9442	0.37	0.7114	0.67	0.5029	0.97	0.3320
0.08	0.9362	0.38	0.7039	0.68	0.4965	0.98	0.3271
0.09	0.9283	0.39	0.6965	0.69	0.4902	0.99	0.3222
0.10	0.9203	0.40	0.6892	0.70	0.4839	1.00	0.3173
0.11	0.9124	0.41	0.6818	0.71	0.4777	1.01	0.3125
0.12	0.9045	0.42	0.6745	0.72	0.4715	1.02	0.3077
0.13	0.8966	0.43	0.6672	0.73	0.4654	1.03	0.3030
0.14	0.8887	0.44	0.6599	0.74	0.4593	1.04	0.2983
0.15	0.8808	0.45	0.6527	0.75	0.4533	1.05	0.2937
0.16	0.8729	0.46	0.6455	0.76	0.4473	1.06	0.2891
0.17	0.8650	0.47	0.6384	0.77	0.4413	1.07	0.2846
0.18	0.8572	0.48	0.6312	0.78	0.4354	1.08	0.2801
0.19	0.8493	0.49	0.6241	0.79	0.4295	1.09	0.2757
0.20	0.8415	0.50	0.6171	0.80	0.4237	1.10	0.2713
0.21	0.8337	0.51	0.6101	0.81	0.4179	1.11	0.2670
0.22	0.8259	0.52	0.6031	0.82	0.4122	1.12	0.2627
0.23	0.8181	0.53	0.5961	0.83	0.4065	1.13	0.2585
0.24	0.8103	0.54	0.5892	0.84	0.4009	1.14	0.2543
0.25	0.8026	0.55	0.5823	0.85	0.3953	1.15	0.2501
0.26	0.7949	0.56	0.5755	0.86	0.3898	1.16	0.2460
0.27	0.7872	0.57	0.5687	0.87	0.3843	1.17	0.2420
0.28	0.7795	0.58	0.5619	0.88	0.3789	1.18	0.2380
0.29	0.7718	0.59	0.5552	0.89	0.3735	1.19	0.2340
0.30	0.7642	0.60	0.5485	0.90	0.3681	1.20	0.2301

z	P	z	P	z	P	z	P
1.21	0.2263	1.61	0.1074	2.01	0.0444	2.41	0.0160
1.22	0.2225	1.62	0.1052	2.02	0.0434	2.42	0.0155
1.23	0.2187	1.63	0.1031	2.03	0.0424	2.43	0.0151
1.24	0.2150	1.64	0.1010	2.04	0.0414	2.44	0.0147
1.25	0.2113	1.65	0.0989	2.05	0.0404	2.45	0.0143
1.26	0.2077	1.66	0.0969	2.06	0.0394	2.46	0.0139
1.27	0.2041	1.67	0.0949	2.07	0.0385	2.47	0.0135
1.28	0.2005	1.68	0.0930	2.08	0.0375	2.48	0.0131
1.29	0.1971	1.69	0.0910	2.09	0.0366	2.49	0.0128
1.30	0.1936	1.70	0.0891	2.10	0.0357	2.50	0.0124
1.31	0.1902	1.71	0.0873	2.11	0.0349	2.51	0.0121
1.32	0.1868	1.72	0.0854	2.12	0.0340	2.52	0.0117
1.33	0.1835	1.73	0.0836	2.13	0.0332	2.53	0.0114
1.34	0.1802	1.74	0.0819	2.14	0.0324	2.54	0.0111
1.35	0.1770	1.75	0.0801	2.15	0.0316	2.55	0.0108
1.36	0.1738	1.76	0.0784	2.16	0.0308	2.56	0.0105
1.37	0.1707	1.77	0.0767	2.17	0.0300	2.57	0.0102
1.38	0.1676	1.78	0.0751	2.18	0.0293	2.58	0.0099
1.39	0.1645	1.79	0.0735	2.19	0.0285	2.59	0.0096
1.40	0.1615	1.80	0.0719	2.20	0.0278	2.60	0.0093
1.41	0.1585	1.81	0.0703	2.21	0.0271	2.61	0.0091
1.42	0.1556	1.82	0.0688	2.22	0.0264	2.62	0.0088
1.43	0.1527	1.83	0.0672	2.23	0.0257	2.63	0.0085
1.44	0.1499	1.84	0.0658	2.24	0.0251	2.64	0.0083
1.45	0.1471	1.85	0.0643	2.25	0.0244	2.65	0.0080
1.46	0.1443	1.86	0.0629	2.26	0.0238	2.66	0.0078
1.47	0.1416	1.87	0.0615	2.27	0.0232	2.67	0.0076
1.48	0.1389	1.88	0.0601	2.28	0.0226	2.68	0.0074
1.49	0.1362	1.89	0.0588	2.29	0.0220	2.69	0.0071
1.50	0.1336	1.90	0.0574	2.30	0.0214	2.70	0.0069
1.51	0.1310	1.91	0.0561	2.31	0.0209	2.71	0.0067
1.52	0.1285	1.92	0.0549	2.32	0.0203	2.72	0.0065
1.53	0.1260	1.93	0.0536	2.33	0.0198	2.73	0.0063
1.54	0.1236	1.94	0.0524	2.34	0.0193	2.74	0.0061
1.55	0.1211	1.95	0.0512	2.35	0.0188	2.75	0.0060
1.56	0.1188	1.96	0.0500	2.36	0.0183	2.76	0.0058
1.57	0.1164	1.97	0.0488	2.37	0.0178	2.77	0.0056
1.58	0.1141	1.98	0.0477	2.38	0.0173	2.78	0.0054
1.59	0.1118	1.99	0.0466	2.39	0.0168	2.79	0.0053
1.60	0.1096	2.00	0.0455	2.40	0.0164	2.80	0.0051
						2.81	0.0050
						2.82	0.0048
						2.83	0.0047
						2.84	0.0045
						2.85	0.0044
						2.86	0.0042
						2.87	0.0041
						2.88	0.0040
						2.89	0.0039
						2.90	0.0037

z	P	z	P	z	P	z	P
						2.91	0.0036
						2.92	0.0035
						2.93	0.0034
						2.94	0.0033
						2.95	0.0032
						2.96	0.0031
						2.97	0.0030
						2.98	0.0029
						2.99	0.0028
						3.00	0.0027
						3.10	0.00194
						3.20	0.00137
						3.30	0.00097
						3.40	0.00067
						3.50	0.00047
						3.60	0.00032
						3.70	0.00022
						3.80	0.00014
						3.90	0.00010
						4.00	0.00006

THE *T*-DISTRIBUTION (ALTMAN, 1991)
REPRODUCED WITH PERMISSION

Degrees of freedom	Two-tailed probability (*P*)					
	0.2	0.1	0.05	0.02	0.01	0.001
1	3.078	6.314	12.706	31.821	63.657	636.619
2	1.886	2.920	4.303	6.965	9.925	31.599
3	1.638	2.353	3.182	4.541	5.841	12.924
4	1.533	2.132	2.776	3.747	4.604	8.610
5	1.476	2.015	2.571	3.365	4.032	6.869
6	1.440	1.943	2.447	3.143	3.707	5.959
7	1.415	1.895	2.365	2.998	3.499	5.408
8	1.397	1.860	2.306	2.896	3.355	5.041
9	1.383	1.833	2.262	2.821	3.250	4.781
10	1.372	1.812	2.228	2.764	3.169	4.587
11	1.363	1.796	2.201	2.718	3.106	4.437
12	1.356	1.782	2.179	2.681	3.055	4.318
13	1.350	1.771	2.160	2.650	3.012	4.221
14	1.345	1.761	2.145	2.624	2.977	4.140
15	1.341	1.753	2.131	2.602	2.947	4.073
16	1.337	1.746	2.120	2.583	2.921	4.015
17	1.333	1.740	2.110	2.567	2.898	3.965
18	1.330	1.734	2.101	2.552	2.878	3.922
19	1.328	1.729	2.093	2.539	2.861	3.883
20	1.325	1.725	2.086	2.528	2.845	3.850
21	1.323	1.721	2.080	2.518	2.831	3.819
22	1.321	1.717	2.074	2.508	2.819	3.792
23	1.319	1.714	2.069	2.500	2.807	3.768
24	1.318	1.711	2.064	2.492	2.797	3.745
25	1.316	1.708	2.060	2.485	2.787	3.725
26	1.315	1.706	2.056	2.479	2.779	3.707
27	1.314	1.703	2.052	2.473	2.771	3.690
28	1.313	1.701	2.048	2.467	2.763	3.674
29	1.311	1.699	2.045	2.462	2.756	3.659
30	1.310	1.697	2.042	2.457	2.750	3.646
31	1.309	1.696	2.040	2.453	2.744	3.633
32	1.309	1.694	2.037	2.449	2.738	3.622
33	1.308	1.692	2.035	2.445	2.733	3.611
34	1.307	1.691	2.032	2.441	2.728	3.601
35	1.306	1.690	2.030	2.438	2.724	3.591
36	1.306	1.688	2.028	2.434	2.719	3.582
37	1.305	1.687	2.026	2.431	2.715	3.574
38	1.304	1.686	2.024	2.429	2.712	3.566
39	1.304	1.685	2.023	2.426	2.708	3.558
40	1.303	1.684	2.021	2.423	2.704	3.551
41	1.303	1.683	2.020	2.421	2.701	3.544
42	1.302	1.682	2.018	2.418	2.698	3.538
43	1.302	1.681	2.017	2.416	2.695	3.532
44	1.301	1.680	2.015	2.414	2.692	3.526
45	1.301	1.679	2.014	2.412	2.690	3.520

Degrees of freedom	Two-tailed probability (P)					
	0.2	0.1	0.05	0.02	0.01	0.001
46	1.300	1.679	2.013	2.410	2.687	3.515
47	1.300	1.678	2.012	2.408	2.685	3.510
48	1.299	1.677	2.011	2.407	2.682	3.505
49	1.299	1.677	2.010	2.405	2.680	3.500
50	1.299	1.676	2.009	2.403	2.678	3.496
51	1.298	1.675	2.008	2.402	2.676	3.492
52	1.298	1.675	2.007	2.400	2.674	3.488
53	1.298	1.674	2.006	2.399	2.672	3.484
54	1.297	1.674	2.005	2.397	2.670	3.480
55	1.297	1.673	2.004	2.396	2.668	3.476
56	1.297	1.673	2.003	2.395	2.667	3.473
57	1.297	1.672	2.002	2.394	2.665	3.470
58	1.296	1.672	2.002	2.392	2.663	3.466
59	1.296	1.671	2.001	2.391	2.662	3.463
60	1.296	1.671	2.000	2.390	2.660	3.460
70	1.294	1.667	1.994	2.381	2.648	3.435
80	1.292	1.664	1.990	2.374	2.639	3.416
90	1.291	1.662	1.987	2.368	2.632	3.402
100	1.290	1.660	1.984	2.364	2.626	3.390
110	1.289	1.659	1.982	2.361	2.621	3.381
120	1.289	1.658	1.980	2.358	2.617	3.373
130	1.288	1.657	1.978	2.355	2.614	3.367
140	1.288	1.656	1.977	2.353	2.611	3.361
150	1.287	1.655	1.976	2.351	2.609	3.357

THE CHI-SQUARED (χ^2) DISTRIBUTION (ALTMAN, 1991)
REPRODUCED WITH PERMISSION

Degrees of freedom	Two-tailed probability (P)					
	0.2	0.1	0.05	0.02	0.01	0.001
1	1.642	2.706	3.841	5.412	6.635	10.827
2	3.219	4.605	5.991	7.824	9.210	13.815
3	4.642	6.251	7.815	9.837	11.345	16.268
4	5.989	7.779	9.488	11.668	13.277	18.465
5	7.289	9.236	11.070	13.388	15.086	20.517
6	8.558	10.645	12.592	15.033	16.812	22.457
7	9.803	12.017	14.067	16.622	18.475	24.322
8	11.030	13.362	15.507	18.168	20.090	26.125
9	12.242	14.684	16.919	19.679	21.666	27.877
10	13.442	15.987	18.307	21.161	23.209	29.588
11	14.631	17.275	19.675	22.618	24.725	31.264
12	15.812	18.549	21.026	24.054	26.217	32.909
13	16.985	19.812	22.362	25.472	27.688	34.528
14	18.151	21.064	23.685	26.873	29.141	36.123
15	19.311	22.307	24.996	28.259	30.578	37.697
16	20.465	23.542	26.296	29.633	32.000	39.252
17	21.615	24.769	27.587	30.995	33.409	40.790
18	22.760	25.989	28.869	32.346	34.805	42.312
19	23.900	27.204	30.144	33.687	36.191	43.820
20	25.038	28.412	31.410	35.020	37.566	45.315
21	26.171	29.615	32.671	36.343	38.932	46.797
22	27.301	30.813	33.924	37.659	40.289	48.268
23	28.429	32.007	35.172	38.968	41.638	49.728
24	29.553	33.196	36.415	40.270	42.980	51.179
25	30.675	34.382	37.652	41.566	44.314	52.620

Exercises

EXERCISE 1

You are a manager at a large general hospital. A consultant oncologist has approached you to suggest that the hospital allows the use of a costly new drug for the treatment of breast cancer. She refers to a recently published study of the drug. In the study, patients were randomised to receive either the new drug or a standard treatment. Mortality was recorded within the first year and then in the subsequent 2 years. The authors calculated a relative risk for mortality for the new drug compared with standard treatment.

The results of the study showed the relative risk of death in the first year to be 0.75 when comparing the new drug with standard treatment. The relative risk for death up to 3 years was 0.82.

a What is a relative risk and how is it calculated?
b Interpret the above relative risk values.
c List up to three other aspects you might wish to consider before deciding whether or not to allow the use of the new drug.

EXERCISE 2

The results of a trial show that patients from a clinic who were taking a new antihypertensive drug had a mean diastolic blood pressure of 79.2 mmHg (standard error = 1.9), while the mean diastolic blood pressure for patients in the same clinic (from data collected over the past 10 years) who were receiving standard treatment was 83.7 mmHg.

a Calculate a z-score and a P-value for these results.
b Is the difference between the two mean blood pressures statistically significant?
c Explain why or why not.

d Calculate a 95% confidence interval for the mean blood pressure with the new drug.

e How would you interpret the results in light of this?

f Briefly discuss whether you think that *P*-values are more useful than confidence intervals.

EXERCISE 3

In total, 109 men were studied in order to investigate a possible association between alcohol consumption and gastric cancer. Two groups of patients were studied. One group of men who had been newly diagnosed with gastric cancer at three general hospitals was compared with another group randomly selected from male patients who had attended a range of surgical outpatient clinics during the same period. Each patient was asked about their history of alcohol consumption, and was categorised according to their weekly alcohol consumption. High alcohol consumption was defined as more than 28 units per week.

a What type of study was this?

b What are the advantages of this type of study?

c What are the disadvantages of this type of study?

d What confounding factors might be present?

It was found that 35 men had consumed more than 28 units of alcohol per week. A total of 54 men had gastric cancer, 22 of whom had a high alcohol intake.

e Construct a suitable table displaying the results of this study.

f What is the most appropriate measure of association for this situation?

g Calculate the measure of association for this study.

h Interpret this result.

i Does this study prove that high alcohol consumption causes gastric cancer?

EXERCISE 4

Over lunch one day, a cardiologist colleague tells you that he is concerned that several of his patients who are taking a brand new drug for hyperlipidaemia are at increased risk of developing non-Hodgkin's lymphoma. He says that several of his patients on another treatment (with certain similarities, which was introduced 5 years ago) have developed lymphoma, and he is concerned that patients who are taking the new preparation may suffer a similar fate. There is no trial evidence to support this claim, from either before or since the time when the new drug was licensed. Your colleague is interested in conducting some type of study to monitor his own patients who will be taking this new drug over the next couple of years, and he asks your advice about what to do.

a   Suggest a suitable type of study to investigate this.
b   What are the advantages of this type of study?
c   What problems might you experience with this type of study?
d   What confounding factors might you encounter?
e   How could you minimise the effect of these?
f   When you have data from the study, what measure of association would you normally use?
g   Explain what this measure of association means.
h   What method might you use to examine the level of statistical significance?
i   If a strong association and/or statistical significance is reached, would this mean that the new drug causes lymphoma? How can causal relationships be established?

EXERCISE 5

You are working for the health authority in a district called Wellsville, where the director of public health is concerned that the death rate for females aged 35–64 years seems to be very high. You have been asked to investigate this.

You have access to local population figures and data on death rates in the standard population. All data are available categorised into age groups of 35–44, 45–54 and 55–64 years. These data are shown following. You also know that the **total** number of deaths for women aged 35–64 years in Wellsville is 482.

You decide to apply death rates for three women's age groups in the standard population to the age structure for local women in the same age groups, in order to produce a standardised measure of death.

Age-specific death rates for all women in standard population

Age group (years)	Death rate
35–44	0.00076
45–54	0.0032
55–64	0.0083

Population of women aged 35–64 years in Wellsville

Age group (years)	Population
35–44	32 000
45–54	27 400
55–64	23 900

a What type of standardisation is described here?
b Use the provided data to work out the total number of expected deaths in Wellsville, and state these for each of the three age groups.
c Calculate an appropriate standardised death rate measure for Wellsville.
d What is this measure called?
e What conclusions can you draw from this with regard to the local death rate?
f Work out a 95% confidence interval around this measure. What conclusions can you draw from this?
g Perform a test of statistical significance on the measure. What does this actually test with regard to the standardised death rate measure you have calculated? What is the z-score? Does this appear to be statistically significant?
h Does the result obtained from (g) change your conclusions? Why or why not?

EXERCISE 6

A recent study compared post-operative infection rates for a standard orthopaedic procedure with those for a new procedure. The study protocol claimed that roughly equal numbers of patients from 20 preoperative assessment clinics were to be randomly allocated to undergo either the new treatment or the standard procedure.

a What type of study is described here?
b What are the main advantages of this type of study?

In each clinic, the first 20 patients received the new treatment, while the next 20 patients were allocated the standard procedure.

c Comment on this allocation procedure.
d What effect might this allocation procedure have on the results of the study?

The results of the study showed that 48 out of 200 patients who underwent the standard procedure developed an infection, while 32 out of 200 patients who received the new procedure developed an infection.

e Calculate an appropriate measure of association for these results.

f   What is your interpretation of this?

g   What test could you use to find out whether the association is statistically significant?

h   Calculate the appropriate test statistic and *P*-value.

i   Calculate the number needed to treat.

j   What does the figure for the number needed to treat that you have calculated mean?

k   Taking your previous answers into account, do you feel that the new procedure is really better than the standard procedure?

EXERCISE 7

Your local health authority has been approached by a manufacturer which has developed a simple screening test for prostate cancer. The test involves taking a sample of blood which is sent away to the local district hospital's pathology department, and results are available within 5 working days. Each test costs £6.87. The health authority is considering offering this test to all male residents aged over 50 years as part of a screening programme, and has asked you to advise them on whether or not to adopt it.

You contact the manufacturer to request data on its efficacy, and you duly receive an unpublished paper containing the following table:

	Prostate cancer?		
	Yes	No	Total
Positive	572	67	639
Negative	29	4983	5012
Total	601	5050	5651

Result of test (left label for Positive/Negative/Total rows)

a   Calculate the sensitivity of the test. What does this mean?

b   Calculate its specificity. What does this mean?

c   Calculate its positive predictive value. What does this mean?

d   Calculate its negative predictive value. What does this mean?

e   What do you think of the accuracy of this test?

f   How does it match up to each of the four criteria for a screening test?

g   Would you recommend that your health authority adopts this screening programme and test?

EXERCISE 8

The Quality and Outcomes Framework (QOF) is a voluntary reward and incentive programme for general practice in the UK (Health & Social Care Information Centre

2015). Information is gathered on a range of clinical and non-clinical indicators and a number of QOF points are awarded, according to whether or not particular standards have been achieved. A colleague has suggested that the quality of medical services provided (using the number of QOF points as an indicator) is related to the number of patients registered at a practice (list size). To test this, we shall use the null hypothesis that in the population of practices there is no correlation between the number of QOF points achieved and list size.

The following data are collected from 10 randomly selected local practices:

Total QOF points achieved	List size
923	5385
918	1995
1040	9809
983	2038
1038	15300
1049	13618
1048	9222
884	2387
1045	12463
879	2845

a Plot the data onto a suitable graph – what type of correlation do you think applies here?

The data are entered into a computer database, and the following output is produced:

Correlations

		Total QOF points	List size
Total QOF points	Pearson correlation	1	.844**
	Sig. (2-tailed)		.002
	N	10	10
List size	Pearson correlation	.844**	1
	Sig. (2-tailed)	.002	
	N	10	10

**Correlation is significant at the 0.01 level (2-tailed)

Coefficients*

Model	Unstandardized coefficients		Standardized coefficients	t	Sig.
	B	Std. error	Beta		
1 (Constant)	892.605	23.671		37.708	.000
List size	.012	.003	.844	4.454	.002

* Dependent variable: Total QOF points.

b What is the value of r?

c How would you rate the strength of association?

d Is there a significant correlation between QOF score and list size? What is the P-value?

e Do you think that the null hypothesis (that there is no correlation between the number of QOF points achieved and list size) is correct?

f Calculate r^2. What does this mean?

g Calculate the predicted QOF score for practices with list sizes of 5000, 8000 and 10 000.

EXERCISE 9

a Read the following, and identify the type of study, and which type of **bias** is associated with each study.

1. A study of patients with oesophageal cancer: cases are interviewed in hospital and controls at home.

2. A questionnaire is sent to all men over 65. It includes questions about diet, health and physical activity. The intention is to estimate the amount of physical disability in the over 65s.

3. In a study of a new drug treatment, the first 20 patients arriving in clinic are allocated to the new treatment and the next 20 continue with their existing treatment.

4. In total, 1000 coffee drinkers and 1000 non-coffee drinkers are followed up for 10 years to see if they develop pancreatic cancer. At the end of the study, 2% of the 800 coffee drinkers who are still traceable have pancreatic cancer, and 1% of the 900 non-coffee drinkers traced have pancreatic cancer.

b List any possible **confounders** for each of the following studies, and also consider how you could **control** for them.

1. Whether exercise level protects against myocardial infarction.

2. Whether alcohol consumption by expectant mothers causes birth deformities.

3. Whether parental smoking causes asthma.

4. Whether drinking Italian coffee protects against bowel cancer.

c Identify each of the following types of epidemiological study.

1. A study asked a sample of 200 people who were suffering from hepatitis and a further 400 similar people who did **not** have hepatitis about their diet over the past year, especially with regard to consumption of seafood.

2. The health of 100 people who had been exposed to asbestos and 100 people with no such exposure was studied for a period of 5 years.

3. A questionnaire was sent to all residents in a district, asking whether they suffered from diabetes. It also invited them to give other information about their age, sex, ethnic and socio-economic groups, smoking and lifestyle.

4. The notes of 10 patients who had taken a new drug for inflammatory bowel disease were examined, to evaluate the drug's efficacy and document any side effects.

5. A total of 1300 patients suffering from Alzheimer's disease were randomly chosen to receive a new drug, 'Alzaferon', over a period of 3 months. A further 1300 patients with Alzheimer's disease were randomly chosen to receive a standard treatment.

6. A number of personnel standing in a busy shopping centre each stopped 50 women with young children over the course of a weekday, and asked them to answer a short questionnaire about exercise patterns.

7. A total of 500 patients taking a new drug for high cholesterol, plus 500 patients taking a standard treatment, 'Voxostatin', were studied for a period. After 2 weeks, the patients swapped over to the other treatment for a further 2 weeks. Allocation to original treatment groups was done randomly.

EXERCISE 10

A study is being planned to evaluate a new analgesic drug for a particular disease. The aim of the treatment is to reduce the pain score on a standard pain scale, where the highest pain has a score of 30. Statistical analysis will use independent t-tests for two independent groups (patients receiving the new treatment vs. current treatment). A recently published paper reported a mean score of 16.3 in people with the disease who receive the current best treatment, with a standard deviation of 11.4. It is agreed that the smallest effect considered to be clinically important is a **reduction of 2** – or a mean pain score of 14.3.

Calculate the sample size required for the study, assuming a significance level of 0.05 and a power of 80%.

EXERCISE 11

A study examined the healing times in days for the treatment of venous leg ulcers with a new kind of compression bandaging therapy, compared to an accepted standard treatment.

Of 60 patients with venous leg ulcers in a leading teaching hospital, equal numbers of patients were randomly allocated to treatment groups 1 or 2.

Patients in group 1 received the new therapy, while those in group 2 received the standard treatment. The patients were followed up for 3 months.

An independent t-test was used to compare mean healing times between the two groups, and the result was statistically significant (d.f. = 58, $t = -5.965$, $P < 0.001$).

The following are part of the output produced:

Descriptive statistics

Group			
Healing time	1	Mean	36.83
		Std. deviation	7.34
		Minimum	22
		Maximum	55
		N	30
	2	Mean	50.13
		Std. deviation	9.76
		Minimum	23
		Maximum	77
		N	30

Tests of normality

		Kolmogorov–Smirnov			Shapiro–Wilk		
	Group	Statistic	df	Sig.	Statistic	df	Sig.
Healing time	1	.101	30	.200	.973	30	.614
	2	.135	30	.169	.953	30	.202

a Were the data normally distributed? How do you know this?
b Calculate the effect size for this study.
c Comment on the effect size and how it should be interpreted.
d Overall do you think that the new treatment is worthwhile?

EXERCISE 12

Let's finish with 30 questions to test your knowledge of some statistical and epidemiological topics. Very few calculations are required here, and you can find all the answers in the next section.

1. The statement 'The number of MMR vaccinations carried out at Hill View Medical Centre increased by 20% last year' is an example of which kind of statistic?
   a Alpha
   b Descriptive
   c Estimation
   d Inferential
   e None of the above

2. Height is an example of which type of data?
   a Categorical
   b Continuous numerical
   c Dichotomous
   d Ordinary
   e Qualitative

3. Which of the following is true? A P-value of 0.005 means that:
   a a one-tailed hypothesis has been used
   b the exposure has caused the outcome of interest
   c the null hypothesis is true
   d the result is non-significant at the $P < 0.05$ level
   e the result is significant at the $P < 0.05$ level

4. In what circumstances are the mean, median and mode of a dataset equal to one another?
   a When random sampling has been used
   b When the data are bimodal
   c When the data are normally distributed
   d When the data are positively skewed
   e When the null hypothesis is rejected

5. You have been asked to present a frequency distribution of data on diastolic blood pressure in hypertensive patients. Which of the following would be most suitable?
   a A box plot
   b A histogram
   c A line chart
   d A pie chart
   e A regression line

6. What is the probability of throwing a four on a die?
   a   0.00037
   b   0.0333
   c   0.1667
   d   0.8333
   e   1.0

7. Which of the following is true? A standard deviation:
   a   adjusts for differences in age and sex structures between two populations
   b   indicates the difference between a group of values and their mean
   c   is not influenced by extreme values
   d   shows the value of a significant difference between two populations
   e   tests for association between two categorical variables

8. The standard error of a data set will always be:
   a   equal to 1.96 standard deviations
   b   equal to 2.53 standard deviations
   c   heterogeneous
   d   larger than the standard deviation
   e   smaller than the standard deviation

9. Which type of distribution applies to rare events happening randomly over time in a large population?
   a   Binomial
   b   Chi-squared
   c   Normal
   d   Poisson
   e   Student's t

10. Sex is an example of which type of data?
    a   Categorical
    b   Continuous
    c   Discrete numerical
    d   Ordinal
    e   Ratio

11. Which of the following is true? Dichotomous variables:
    a   are negatively skewed
    b   can take any number of possible categories
    c   can take a range of whole numbers
    d   can take one of only two possible categories
    e   none of the above

12. What percentage of values lie within ±1.96 standard deviations of the mean?
    a 0.05
    b 0.95
    c 1.96
    d 95
    e 99.73

13. The following graph is an example of which kind of data?

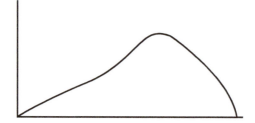

    a Bimodal
    b Binomially distributed
    c Negatively skewed
    d Normally distributed
    e Positively skewed

14. Which of the following is true? Data that are described as 'heterogeneous' are:
    a confounders
    b exactly the same as each other
    c relatively dissimilar to each other
    d relatively similar to each other
    e significantly associated

15. Which of the following is true? Calculating the square root of the variance produces:
    a the arithmetic mean
    b the specificity
    c the squared deviation
    d the standard deviation
    e the standard error

16. Which of the following is true? Parametric tests are carried out on data that are:
    a categorical
    b heterogeneous
    c homogenous
    d non-normally distributed
    e normally distributed

17–19. A dataset consists of the following values:

34	34	35	36	37	38	38
39	40	40	41	41	41	42
44	45	45	46	47	48	48

Calculate the following:

17. _____ the mean (to three decimal places)

18. _____ the median

19. _____ the mode

20. What is the principal type of bias that affects case–control studies?
   a Follow-up bias
   b Interviewer bias
   c Recall bias
   d Selection bias
   e Social acceptability bias

21. What type of bias is represented by the following statement?
   'Patients from socioeconomically deprived groups are less likely to attend for
      subsequent health checks.'
   a Follow-up bias
   b Interviewer bias
   c Misclassification bias
   d Recall bias
   e Social acceptability bias

22. Which is most appropriate to compare death rates between a local population
   and the standard population?
   a Crude death rate
   b Directly standardised death rate
   c Point prevalence
   d Proportional mortality ratio
   e Standardised mortality ratio

For questions 23 and 24:
One method of standardisation typically applies death rates for each age group in the
standard population to the same groups in the local population. An 'expected rate' is
calculated, which is then divided by the observed death rate and multiplied by 100 to
produce a standardised mortality ratio (SMR).

23. What kind of standardisation is described here?
    a   Cohen's standardisation
    b   Direct standardisation
    c   Indirect standardisation
    d   Relative standardisation
    e   Spatial standardisation

24. If a an SMR of 187 is calculated for the situation, this means that:
    a   the death rate in the standard population is 87% higher than the local population
    b   the age-standardised death rate in the local population is 87% higher than the standard population
    c   the age-standardised death rate in the local population is 187% higher than the standard population
    d   the age-standardised death rate in the standard population is 87% higher than the local population
    e   the age-standardised death rate in the standard population is 187% higher than the local population

25. When calculating a sample size, α is usually set at what level?
    a   5%
    b   20%
    c   75%
    d   80%
    e   95%

26. The formula $\dfrac{\text{Disease incidence in exposed group}}{\text{Disease incidence in non-exposed group}}$ represents:

    a   absolute risk
    b   incidence
    c   number needed to treat
    d   odds ratio
    e   relative risk

27. Systematic differences in the way in which subjects are recruited into different groups for a study is an example of:
    a   allocation bias
    b   follow-up bias
    c   recall bias
    d   recording bias
    e   responder bias

28. What do we call the situation where a separate factor (or factors) influences the occurrence of disease, other than the risk factor being studied?
    a   Absolute risk
    b   Causation
    c   Confounding
    d   Modification bias
    e   Validity

29. In screening, the formula $d/(b + d)$ represents:
    a   absolute risk
    b   attributable risk
    c   odds ratio
    d   positive predictive value
    e   specificity

30. Which statistic is commonly used to calculate effect size?
    a   Altman's nomogram
    b   Cohen's d
    c   Fisher's exact test
    d   Shapiro–Wilk test
    e   standardised mortality ratio

Answers to exercises

EXERCISE 1

a A relative risk (or RR) indicates the risk of developing a disease in a group of people who were exposed to a risk factor, relative to a group who were not exposed to it.

It is calculated as follows:

$$RR = \frac{\text{Disease incidence in exposed group}}{\text{Disease incidence in non-exposed group}}$$

Or, using a 2 × 2 table:

$$\frac{a/a+b}{c/c+d}$$

b The relative risks mean that patients who are receiving the new drug are less likely to die at 1 and 3 years. Mortality was reduced by 25% in the first year and by 18% at up to 3 years.

c These could include looking for other studies on the same drug, to check whether they showed different results. Better still, look for a meta-analysis or systematic review, which would combine the results of other studies to produce an overall (and more precise) result. Find out whether any new trials are expected to begin or end in the near future. Is longer-term follow-up planned for any studies? What side effects are associated with the new drug? Have economic considerations such as cost-effectiveness and quality of life been studied?

EXERCISE 2

a $z = (\bar{x} - \mu)/\text{s.e.} = (79.2 - 83.7)/1.9 = 2.37$.

Using the normal distribution table, a z-score of 2.37 produces a P-value of **0.0178**.

b The difference between the two mean values is statistically significant.

c Because the P-value is less than 0.05 (< 0.05 being the usual threshold of statistical significance).

d 95% c.i. $= \bar{x} \pm 1.96 \times \text{s.e.} = 79.2 \pm (1.96 \times 1.9)$

$= 79.2 \pm 3.72 = \textbf{75.5} \rightarrow \textbf{82.9}$ (to one decimal place).

e The confidence interval shows that the true diastolic blood pressure in the population lies between 75.5 and 82.9, with a 95% degree of certainty. The confidence interval is quite narrow. The upper limit does not quite reach the mean for patients receiving standard treatment (83.7), but comes quite close to it. Some caution is therefore suggested.

f P-values only show whether a result is statistically significant, whereas confidence intervals show where the true value lies in the population with 95% confidence, and also indicate significance if the limits do not cross the value with which the sample value is being compared. The confidence interval arguably gives more information; it is useful to present it in combination with a P-value.

EXERCISE 3

a This is a case–control study.

b It is quicker and cheaper than a cohort study, especially suitable for rare diseases, allows investigation of more than one risk factor and is useful for diseases with long latent periods.

c The data are retrospective, so are prone to both selection and information biases. It is difficult to establish the time between exposure and development of disease. Subjects do not usually represent the population as a whole, so incidence rates cannot be calculated, and it is not possible to examine the relationships between one possible cause and several diseases.

d Confounding factors include age, diet, ethnic group, smoking and socio-economic class.

e

		Gastric cancer?		
		Yes	No	Total
High alcohol consumption	**Positive**	22 (a)	13 (b)	35
	Negative	32 (c)	42 (d)	74
	Total	54	55	109

f Odds ratio.

g Odds ratio = $(a/c)/(b/d)$ = $(22/32)/(13/42)$ = $0.6875/0.3095$ = **2.22**.

h Men with alcohol consumption of over 28 units per week are 2.22 times more likely to develop gastric cancer than those whose weekly consumption is 28 units or less.

i No. It is possible that other factors may have been responsible for the gastric cancer, so more research is needed to establish causality.

EXERCISE 4

a Cohort study.

b It allows outcomes to be explored over time, the incidence of disease in both exposed and non-exposed groups can be measured, it is useful for rare exposures, it can examine the effects of more than one exposure, and it is more representative of the true population than case–control studies.

c It can take a very long time to complete, diseases with long latent periods may need many years of follow-up, it is not so useful for rare diseases, it can be very expensive, and careful follow-up of all subjects is vital.

d Possible confounders include age, sex, ethnic group, smoking status and socio-economic status.

e Use stratification, matching and random selection of subjects.

f Relative risk is normally used.

g The risk of developing a disease in a group of people who were exposed to a risk factor, relative to a group who were not exposed to it.

h Methods of examining statistical significance include hypothesis (e.g. normal test or t-tests) and Chi-squared tests.

i Not necessarily – the disease could be caused by other factors, and this possibility merits further investigation. If other possible factors and potential causes can be eliminated (including chance findings, biases and confounders), the presence of the following can provide strong evidence of causality: dose–response, strength, disease specificity, time relationship, biological plausibility and consistency (*see* Chapter 26).

EXERCISE 5

a Indirect standardisation.

b 35–44 years $(0.00076 \times 32\,000) = 24.32$
    45–54 years $(0.0032 \times 27\,400) = 87.68$
    55–64 years $(0.0083 \times 23\,900) = 198.37$
    Expected number of deaths = $24.32 + 87.68 + 198.37 = 310.37$.

c SMR = (observed deaths/expected deaths) $\times$ 100

Observed deaths = 482   Expected deaths = 310.37

Therefore SMR = (482/310.37) × 100 = **155**.

d Standardised mortality ratio or SMR.

e The Wellsville death rate is 55% higher than that of the standard population.

f First calculate the standard error (s.e.) for the SMR, and then work out the confidence interval:

$$s.e. = \left(\frac{\sqrt{O}}{E}\right) \times 100$$

where O = observed deaths and E = expected deaths.

So

$$s.e. = \left(\frac{\sqrt{482}}{310.37}\right) \times 100 = \left(\frac{21.954}{310.37}\right) \times 100 = 7.073$$

95% c.i. = 155 ± (1.96 × 7.073) = 155 ± 13.863.

95% c.i. 155 (141.137 → 168.863) or, using whole numbers, 155 (141 → 169).

The confidence interval does not span 100 and is arguably not too wide. The Wellsville SMR appears to differ significantly from that of the standard population.

g $z = (O - E)/\sqrt{E}\ ) = (482 - 310.37)/\sqrt{310.37}\ = (482 - 310.37)/17.617 = 171.63/17.617$ = 9.74:

This tests the null hypothesis that the SMR for Wellsville = 100.

Using the normal distribution table, a z-score of 9.74 produces a P-value of < 0.00006 (the highest z-value covered by the normal distribution table in this book is 4.00), which is significant. We can reject the null hypothesis that Wellsville's SMR = 100, and thus the alternative hypothesis that the SMR is different.

h No. The 95% confidence interval also indicates significance.

EXERCISE 6

a This is a randomised controlled trial (RCT).

b It allows the effectiveness of a new treatment to be evaluated, it provides strong evidence of effectiveness, and it is less prone to confounding than other study designs.

c Possible biases include the following. The patients were not randomly allocated – using the first 20 patients is biased, as these patients could have arrived first because they were least ill or most ill, they could have been private patients, or they could have arrived early because they used hospital transport due to inability to travel independently. Selecting patients in this way means that they could have been systematically different to the controls.

d This could invalidate the results of the trial – this 'RCT' is not randomised!

e

		Infection?		
		Yes	No	Total
Which procedure?	**New**	32 (*a*)	168 (*b*)	200 (*a* + *b*)
	Standard	48 (*c*)	152 (*d*)	200 (*c* + *d*)
	Total	80 (*a* + *c*)	320 (*b* + *d*)	400 (*a* + *b* + *c* + *d*)

The appropriate measure is relative risk.

$$RR = \frac{a/a+b}{c/c+d} = \frac{32/200}{48/200} = \frac{0.16}{0.24} = 0.67.$$

f Patients undergoing the new procedure are 33% less likely to get a post-operative infection than those undergoing the standard procedure.

g Chi-squared test.

h Work out the expected frequencies for each cell:

cell a: $[(a + b) \times (a + c)/\text{total}] = (200 \times 80)/400 = 40.$
cell b: $[(a + b) \times (b + d)/\text{total}] = (200 \times 320)/400 = 160.$
cell c: $[(a + c) \times (c + d)/\text{total}] = (80 \times 200)/400 = 40.$
cell d: $[(b + d) \times (c + d)/\text{total}] = (320 \times 200)/400 = 160.$

	O	*E*	(*O* − *E*)	(*O* − *E*)^2	[(*O* − *E*)^2/*E*]
a	32	40	−8	64	1.60
b	168	160	8	64	0.40
c	48	40	8	64	1.60
d	152	160	−8	64	0.40
Total	400				4.00

The value of χ^2 is 4.0 and d.f. = 1. Use the Chi-squared distribution table to look up the *P*-value. The *P*-value is < 0.05, which is statistically significant.

To work out χ^2 with Yates' correction:

	O	*E*	[I(*O* − *E*)I− 0.5]	[I(*O* − *E*)I− 0.5]^2	[(I(*O* − *E*)I− 0.5)^2/*E*]
a	32	40	7.5	56.25	1.41
b	168	160	7.5	56.25	0.35
c	48	40	7.5	56.25	1.41
d	152	160	7.5	56.25	0.35
Total	400				3.52

Using Yates' correction produces a χ^2 value of 3.52. *P* is now > 0.05, which is **not** statistically significant.

i   NNT = 24% − 16% = 8%. 100/8 = **12.5** or 13 (rounded to nearest whole number).

j   Around 13 patients will need to be treated with the new procedure in order to prevent one additional infection.

k   The new procedure does not appear to be significantly better than the standard procedure. Although RR = 0.67, representing a 33% reduction in risk, the Chi-squared test with Yates' correction is not significant. The NNT is fairly high. Also remember that treatment allocation was not random.

EXERCISE 7

a   Sensitivity = $a/(a + c)$ = 572/601 = **0.952** or 95.2%. This is the proportion of subjects who really have the disease, and who have been identified as diseased by the test.

b   Specificity = $d/(b + d)$ = 4983/5050 = **0.987** or 98.7%. This is the proportion of subjects who really do not have the disease, and who have been identified as disease-free by the test.

c   PPV = $a/(a + b)$ = 572/639 = **0.895** or 89.5%. This is the probability that a subject with a positive test result really does have the disease.

d   NPV = $d/(c + d)$ = 4983/5012 = **0.994** or 99.4%. This is the probability that a subject with a negative test result really does not have the disease.

e   The overall accuracy is good, although the PPV is only 89.5%; 100% cannot be realistically achieved; false-positives and false negatives are low.

f   It seems to be simple, safe and acceptable. The health authority has not commented on the distribution of test values and cut-off levels, or agreed a policy on further investigations of subjects with a positive result or what their choices might be – these items require agreement and clarification. However, the low PPV could indicate problems with precision. Also see answer to (g).

g   Although the test sounds reasonable on the basis of the study provided, further evidence is required before the screening programme should be adopted. The study supplied by the manufacturer is unpublished – this may indicate that it has not been considered to be of high enough quality for publication. It would be worthwhile searching for other published and unpublished material, and seeking further details from the manufacturer. The test should be compared with alternative screening programmes. Even if strong evidence of the test's accuracy is established, the health authority will of course need to consider all of the UK National Screening Committee's criteria and make the appropriate arrangements before implementing the programme.

EXERCISE 8

a Imperfect positive correlation – see graph:

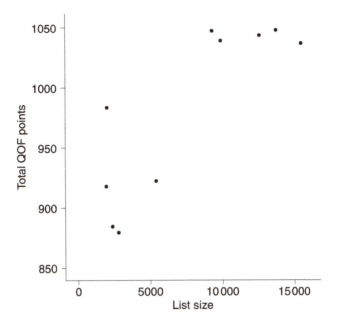

b $r = 0.844$.

c Very strong.

d Yes, there is a significant correlation between QOF score and list size.
The P-value is shown as 0.002 on the computer output.

e No, the significant P-value does not support the null hypothesis, which can be
rejected. We are, of course, assuming that QOF points are an accurate indicator of
practice quality.

f $r^2 = 0.712$. This means that list size is responsible for 71.2% of the total variation
in QOF score.

g This is calculated using linear regression. The formula for the regression line is:
$y = a + bx$. In this example:

y = Total QOF points
x = List size
$a = 892.605$
$b = 0.012$

So: Total QOF points = 892.605 + (0.012 × List size)
For a list size of 5000:
Total QOF points = 892.605 + (0.012 × List size)
i.e. Total QOF points = 892.605 + (0.012 × 5000)

i.e. Total QOF points = 892.605 + 60
i.e. Total QOF points = **952.605** (or **953** to the nearest whole number)

So a practice with a list size of 5000 would be predicted to achieve **953** QOF points.

For a list size of 8000:
Total QOF points = 892.605 + (0.012 × List size)
i.e. Total QOF points = 892.605 + (0.012 × 8000)
i.e. Total QOF points = 892.605 + 96
i.e. Total QOF points = **988.605** (or **989** to the nearest whole number)

So a practice with a list size of 8000 would be predicted to achieve **989** QOF points.

For a list size of 10 000:
Total QOF points = 892.605 + (0.012 × List size)
i.e. Total QOF points = 892.605 + (0.012 × 10 000)
i.e. Total QOF points = 892.605 + 120
i.e. Total QOF points = **1012.605** (or **1013** to the nearest whole number)

So a practice with a list size of 10 000 would be predicted to achieve **1013** QOF points.

EXERCISE 9

a Answers include:
1. Case–control study. **Selection and information biases**, but **recall bias** is a particular problem for case–control studies.
2. Cross-sectional study. **Selection (responder) bias**. A written questionnaire means that disabled people may be less able to respond. Disability is often seen as a stigma which people may not wish to admit to. Alternatively, they may over-estimate their disability, e.g. if they hope to get a car sticker for access to disabled parking.
3. Intervention study. **Selection bias**. Early arrivals may be fitter, wealthier (not reliant on public transport), type A personality. Or the consultant may have asked for sicker patients to be given the earlier appointments.
4. Cohort study. **Follow-up bias**.
b Answers include:
1. Whether exercise level protects against myocardial infarction: *smoking, sex, age*.
2. Whether alcohol consumption by expectant mothers causes birth deformities: *smoking, age, drug use, alcohol, genetics*.

3. Whether parental smoking causes asthma:
   damp housing, genetics, environmental pollutants.
4. Whether drinking Italian coffee protects against bowel cancer:
   diet, including consumption of fresh fruit and vegetables, alcohol consumption, genetics.

Control measures include:
- **randomisation** – in intervention studies
- **restricting admissibility criteria** – e.g. men only, hence sex cannot confound. Cheap and simple but reduces the number of eligible subjects; reduced generalisability; does not restrict other confounders
- **matching** – difficult, costly and time-consuming. Lose potential subjects; only controls matched factors; can't evaluate influence of matched factor
- **stratified analysis.**

c
1. Case–control study
2. Prospective cohort study
3. Cross-sectional (prevalence) study
4. Case series
5. Randomised controlled trial
6. Survey with quota sampling
7. Randomised controlled cross-over trial

EXERCISE 10

Using Altman's nomogram

The first step is to calculate the **standardised difference**. This is the effect being studied (difference in pain scores), divided by the SD.

The standardised difference is calculated as: 2/11.4 = **0.18** (actually 0.175)

We want to use a significance level of **0.05**, and power of **0.8**.

To find the sample size on the nomogram:

- make a line from 0.175 on the standardised difference line (down the left-hand side) to 0.8 on the power line (down the right-hand side)
- read off the total sample size along the 0.05 significance level line.

As shown in the nomogram following, this crosses the 0.05 line at around 1000, indicating that approximately 500 patients will be needed for each group.

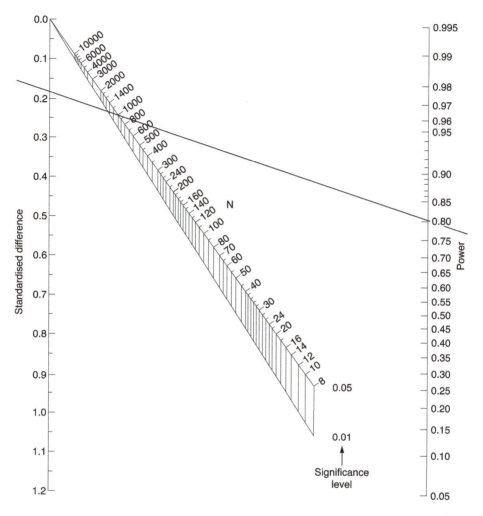

Using the online calculator

After accessing the online sample size calculator, select the second option 'Comparing Means for Two Independent Samples', then:

- type in the score on pain scale (with current treatment) into **mu1** – 16.3
- type in the score on pain scale (expected with new treatment) into **mu2** – 14.3
- type the SD into **sigma** – 11.4
- click 'Calculate'.

The sample size for each group is **511**.

The online calculator readout is shown following.

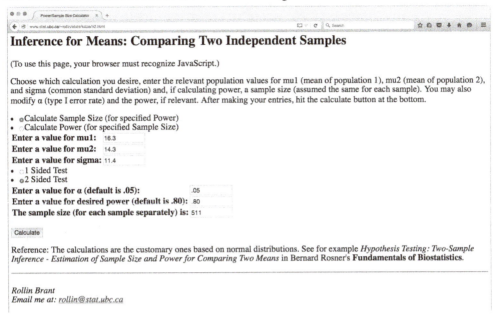

EXERCISE 11

a   Yes, the data can reasonably be assumed to be normally distributed. As the sample size was less than 50 for each group, the Shapiro–Wilk test should be used for each variable. For group 1, the Shapiro–Wilk significance was 0.614, and for group 2 it was 0.202. As these are both > 0.05, normality can be assumed.

b   To calculate Cohen's d, we need the following information:

Mean of group 1 = 36.83   SD of group 1 = 7.34
Mean of group 2 = 50.13   SD of group 2 = 9.76

If we use the control group SD (group 2 = 9.76), Cohen's d would be calculated as:

$$d = \frac{m_1 - m_2}{SD}$$

$$= \frac{36.83 - 50.13}{SD}$$

$$= \frac{13.3}{SD} \quad \text{(we are only interested in the difference, so ignore the minus value)}$$

$$= \frac{13.3}{9.76}$$

$$= \mathbf{1.36}$$

Because the SDs are different, we could calculate a pooled SD as follows:

$$\text{For pooled SD} = \sqrt{\frac{(SD_1^2 + SD_2^2)}{2}}$$

$$= \sqrt{\frac{(7.34^2 + 9.76^2)}{2}}$$

$$= \sqrt{\frac{(53.88 + 95.26)}{2}}$$

$$= \sqrt{\frac{149.14}{2}}$$

$$= \sqrt{74.57}$$

$$= \mathbf{8.64}$$

To complete our effect size calculation using pooled SD:

$$d = \frac{m_1 - m_2}{SD}$$

$$= \frac{36.83 - 50.13}{SD}$$

$$= \frac{13.3}{SD} \quad \text{(ignoring the minus value)}$$

$$= \frac{13.3}{8.64}$$

$$= \mathbf{1.54}$$

c Going back to our classification of d, both 1.36 and 1.54 are far higher than 0.8, so would be regarded as a large effect size.

d The independent t-test produces a statistically significant result, and a large effect size has been demonstrated. A difference in healing time of 13 days could well be regarded as clinically important. The study was a randomised controlled trial (RCT), which, if well designed and executed may provide strong evidence of effectiveness. Not much information is given, however, on the quality of the RCT (e.g. how randomisation was carried out, whether single or double blinding or intention-to-treat analysis was used). The sample size was relatively small, and we do not know whether an *a priori* sample size calculation was carried out (though you could use the online sample size calculator used in Chapter 21 to calculate a *post-hoc* sample size). It is also unlikely that just one RCT could provide enough evidence to allow a judgement about whether the new treatment is effective and safe.

There is therefore some evidence that the new treatment is worthwhile, but more information and research are required.

EXERCISE 12

1. b. Descriptive
2. b. Continuous numerical
3. e. The result is significant at the $P < 0.05$ level
4. c. When the data are normally distributed
5. b. A histogram
6. c. 0.1667
7. b. Indicates the difference between a group of values and their mean
8. e. Smaller than the standard deviation
9. d. Poisson
10. a. Categorical
11. d. Can take one of only two possible categories
12. d. 95
13. c. Negatively skewed
14. c. Relatively dissimilar to each other
15. d. The standard deviation
16. e. Normally distributed
17.   Mean = 40.905
18.   Median = 41
19.   Mode = 41
20. c. Recall bias
21. a. Follow-up bias
22. e. Standardised mortality ratio
23. c. Indirect standardisation
24. b. The age-standardised death rate in the local population is 87% higher than the standard population
25. a. 5%
26. e. Relative risk
27. a. Allocation bias
28. c. Confounding
29. e. Specificity
30. b. Cohen's *d*

References

Altman DG (1991) *Practical Statistics for Medical Research*. Chapman & Hall, London.

Altman DG (1982) How large a sample? In: SM Gore and DG Altman (eds) *Statistics in Practice*. BMA, London.

Armitage P, Matthews JNS and Berry G (2001) *Statistical Methods in Medical Research* (4e). Blackwell Scientific Publications, Oxford.

Barton B and Peat J (2014) *Medical Statistics: a guide to SPSS, data analysis and critical appraisal* (2e). Wiley, Chichester.

Bland M (2000) *An Introduction to Medical Statistics* (3e). Oxford University Press, Oxford.

Bowling A (1997) *Measuring Health: a review of quality of life measurement scales* (2e). Open University Press, Buckingham.

Bowling A (2001) *Measuring Disease: a review of disease-specific quality of life measurement scales* (2e). Open University Press, Buckingham.

Bowling A (2014) *Research Methods in Health: investigating health and health services* (4e). Open University Press, Maidenhead.

Bradford-Hill AB (1965) The environment and disease: association or causation? *Proc R Soc Med*. **58**: 295–300.

Brant R (2015) [Web-based sample size/power calculations]. Available online at: www.stat.ubc. ca/~rollin/stats/ssize/ (accessed 26/02/2015).

CASP (2013) *10 Questions to Help You Make Sense of a Review*. CASP, Oxford. Available online at: http://media.wix.com/ugd/dded87_a02ff2e3445f4952992d5a96ca562576.pdf (accessed 18/09/2015).

Chen CC, David AS, Nunnerley H *et al.* (1995) Adverse life events and breast cancer: case–control study. *BMJ*. **311**: 1527–30.

Coggon D, Rose G and Barker DJP (1997) *Epidemiology for the Uninitiated* (4e). BMJ Publications, London.

Cohen J (1988) *Statistical Power Analysis for the Behavioural Sciences* (2e). L Erlbaum Associates, Mahwah, NJ.

CONSORT (2010) CONSORT 2010 Statement. CONSORT, Ottawa, ON. Available online at: www. consort-statement.org (accessed 26/02/2015).

Dawes M, Summerskill W, Glasziou P *et al.* (2005) Sicily Statement on evidence-based practice. *BMC Med Educ*. **5**(5): 1.

Department of Public Health and Epidemiology (1999) *Epidemiological Methods 1999*. Department of Public Health and Epidemiology, University of Birmingham, Birmingham.

DiCenso A, Bayley L and Haynes RB (2009) Accessing preappraised evidence: fine tuning the 5S model into a 6S model. *ACP J Club*. **151**(3). Available online at: http://plus.mcmaster.ca/mac plusfs/documentation/Haynes_6S_Editorial.pdf (accessed 18/09/2015).

Donaldson L and Scally G (2009) *Donaldson's Essential Public Health* (3e). Radcliffe Publishing, Oxford.

Donaldson RJ and Donaldson LJ (2000) *Essential Public Health* (2e). Petroc Press, Newbury.

Field A (2013) *Discovering Statistics using IBM SPSS Statistics* (4e). Sage, London.

Freeman P (1997) Mindstretcher: logistic regression explained. *Bandolier*. 37: 5. Available online at: www.medicine.ox.ac.uk/bandolier/band37/b37-5.html (accessed 26/02/2015).

Fritzsche FR, Ramach C, Soldini D *et al.* (2012) Occupational health risks of pathologists – results from a nationwide online questionnaire in Switzerland. *BMC Public Health*. 12: 1054. Available online at: www.biomedcentral.com/1471-2458/12/1054 (accessed 26/02/2015).

Glasziou P, Irwig L, Bain C *et al.* (2001) *Systematic Reviews in Health Care: a practical guide*. Cambridge University Press, Cambridge.

GRADE working group (2015) Grading the quality of evidence and the strength of recommendations. GRADE working group. Available online at: www.gradeworkinggroup.org/intro.htm (accessed 26/02/2015).

Hamberg K J, Carstensen B, Sorensen TI *et al.* (1996) Accuracy of clinical diagnosis of cirrhosis among alcohol-abusing men. *J Clin Epidem*. 49(11): 1295–301.

Harris J (2005) It's not NICE to discriminate. *J Med Ethics*. 31: 373–5.

Health & Social Care Information Centre (HSCIC) (n.d.) Quality and outcomes framework. HSCIC, Leeds. Available online at: www.hscic.gov.uk/qof (accessed 26/02/15).

Hicks N (1997) Evidence based health care. *Bandolier*. 39: 9. Available online at: www.medicine.ox.ac.uk/bandolier/band39/b39-9.html (accessed 20/08/ 2009).

IBM Corporation (2013) IBM SPSS Statistics (Version 22.0) [software]. IBM Corporation, Armonk, NY.

Kirkwood B (1988) *Essentials of Medical Statistics*. Blackwell Scientific Publications, Oxford.

Kirkwood BR and Sterne JAC (2003) *Essential Medical Statistics* (2e). Blackwell Scientific Publications, Oxford.

Last JM (2001) *A Dictionary of Epidemiology* (4e). Oxford University Press, Oxford.

Lewis GH, Sherringham J, Kalim K *et al.* (2008) *Mastering Public Health: a postgraduate guide to examinations and revalidation*. CRC Press, Boca Raton, FL.

Lilienfeld DE and Stolley PD (1994) *Foundations of Epidemiology* (3e). Oxford University Press, Oxford.

Moher D, Liberati A, Tetzlaff J *et al.* for the PRISMA Group (2009) Preferred reporting items for systematic reviews and meta-analyses: the PRISMA Statement. *BMJ*. 339: b2535. (The PRISMA Statement website is online at: www.prisma-statement.org/ (accessed 10/04/2015)).

NHS Health Scotland, University of Warwick and University of Edinburgh (2006) The Warwick-Edinburgh Mental Well-being Scale (WEMWBS). NHS Health Scotland, University of Warwick and University of Edinburgh, Edinburgh. Available online at: www.healthscotland.com/documents/1467.aspx (accessed 07/03/2015).

NICE (2015). [Q section of NICE Glossary]. NICE, London. Available online at: www.nice.org.uk/glossary?letter=q (accessed 11/04/2015).

Orme J, Powell J, Taylor P *et al.* (2003) *Public Health for the 21st Century: new perspectives on policy, participation and practice*. Open University Press, Maidenhead.

Oscier DG (1997) ABC of clinical haematology: the myelodysplastic syndromes. *BMJ*. 314: 883–6.

Petrie A and Sabin C (2009) *Medical Statistics at a Glance* (3e). Wiley-Blackwell, Chichester.

Po ALW (1998) *Dictionary of Evidence-based Medicine*. Radcliffe Medical Press, Oxford.

Ralph SG, Rutherford AJ and Wilson JD (1999) Influence of bacterial vaginosis on conception and miscarriage in the first trimester: cohort study. *BMJ*. 319: 220–3.

Rowntree D (1981) *Statistics Without Tears: a primer for non-mathematicians*. Penguin, Harmondsworth.

Sackett DL, Richardson WS, Rosenberg W *et al.* (1997) *Evidence-Based Medicine. How to practice and teach EBM* (2e). Churchill Livingstone, Edinburgh.

Sackett DL, Straus SE, Richardson WS *et al.* (2000) *Evidence-Based Medicine. How to practice and teach EBM* (2e). Churchill Livingstone, London.

Smeeton N and Goda D (2003) Conducting and presenting social work research: some basic statistical considerations. *Br J Soc Work*. **33**(4): 567–73.

Stewart A (2010) Lifting the fog – bringing clarity to public health. *Perspect Public Health*. **130**(6): 263–4.

Stewart A and Rao JN (2000) Do Asians with diabetes in Sandwell receive inferior primary care? A retrospective cohort study. *J R Soc Promotion Health*. **120**: 248–54.

Swinscow TDV and Campbell MJ (2002) *Statistics at Square One* (10e). BMJ Publications, London.

Tilson JK, Kaplan SL, Harris JL *et al.* (2011) Sicily statement on classification and development of evidence-based practice learning assessment tools. *BMC Med Educ*. **11**: 78. Available online at: www.biomedcentral.com/1472-6920/11/78 (accessed 26/02/2015).

UK National Screening Committee (2015) Programme Appraisal Criteria: criteria for assessing the viability, effectiveness and appropriateness of a screening programme. Available online at: www.screening.nhs.uk/criteria (accessed 26/02/2015). Contains public sector information licensed under the Open Government Licence v3.0. Available online at: www.nationalarchives.gov.uk/doc/open-government-licence/version/3 (accessed 18/09/2015).

Wilson JMG and Jungner G (1968) *Principles and Practice of Screening for Disease*. Public Health Paper Number 34. World Health Organization, Geneva.

World Medical Association (2013) *WMA Declaration of Helsinki – ethical principles for medical research involving human subjects*. Available online at: www.wma.net/en/30publications/10policies/b3/ (accessed 26/02/2015).

Further reading: a selection

Altman DG (1991) *Practical Statistics for Medical Research*. Chapman & Hall, London.

Altman DG, Machin D, Bryant TN *et al.* (2000) *Statistics with Confidence* (2e). BMJ Publishing, London.

Armitage P, Matthews JNS and Berry G (2001) *Statistical Methods in Medical Research* (4e). Blackwell Scientific Publications, Oxford.

Barker DJP, Cooper C and Rose GR (1998) *Epidemiology in Medical Practice* (5e). Churchill Livingstone, Edinburgh.

Ben-Shlomo Y, Brookes S, Hickman M (2013) *Epidemiology, Evidence-based Medicine and Public Health: lecture notes* (6e). Wiley-Blackwell, Chichester.

Bhopal R (2008) *Concepts of Epidemiology* (2e). Oxford University Press, Oxford.

Bland M (2015) *Introduction to Medical Statistics* (4e). Oxford University Press, Oxford.

Bonita R, Beaglehole R and Kjellström T (2006) *Basic Epidemiology* (2e). World Health Organization, Geneva. Available for free download at: apps.who.int/iris/bitstream/10665/43541/1/9241547073_eng.pdf?ua=1 (accessed 18/09/2015).

Borenstein M, Hedges LV, Higgins JPT *et al.* (2009) *Introduction to Meta-analysis*. Wiley-Blackwell, Chichester.

Bowers D (2014) *Medical Statistics from Scratch: an introduction for health care professionals* (3e). Wiley-Blackwell, Chichester.

Bowling A (2014) *Research Methods in Health: investigating health and health services* (4e). Open University Press, Maidenhead.

Campbell MJ (2009) *Statistics at Square One* (11e). Wiley-Blackwell, Chichester.

Carr S, Unwin N and Pless-Mulloli T (2007) *An Introduction to Public Health and Epidemiology* (2e). Open University Press, Maidenhead.

Coggon D, Rose G and Barker DJP (2003) *Epidemiology for the Uninitiated* (5e). BMJ Publications, London.

Cumming G (2012). *Understanding the New Statistics: effect sizes, confidence intervals, and meta-analysis*. Routledge, New York, NY, and Hove.

Donaldson L and Scally G (2009) *Donaldson's Essential Public Health* (3e). Radcliffe Publishing, Oxford.

Field A (2013) *Discovering Statistics using IBM SPSS Statistics* (4e). Sage, London.

Greenhalgh T (2014) *How to Read a Paper: the basics of evidence based medicine* (5e). Wiley-Blackwell, Chichester.

Higgins JPT and Green S (eds) (2011) *Cochrane Handbook for Systematic Reviews of Interventions* (Version 5.1.0) (updated March 2011). Available online at: www.cochrane-handbook.org/ (accessed 8/10/2015).

Kirkwood BR and Sterne JAC (2003) *Essential Medical Statistics* (2e). Wiley-Blackwell, Chichester.

MacDonald TH (2006) *Basic Concepts in Statistics and Epidemiology*. Radcliffe Publishing, Oxford.

Petrie A and Sabin C (2009) *Medical Statistics at a Glance* (3e). Wiley-Blackwell, Chichester (a workbook is also available separately).

Porta M (ed) (2008) *A Dictionary of Epidemiology* (5e). Oxford University Press, Oxford and New York, NY.

Rothman KJ (2012) *Epidemiology: an introduction* (2e). Oxford University Press, New York, NY.

Rothman KJ, Greenland S and Lash TL (2013) *Modern Epidemiology* (3e mid-cycle revision). Lippincott Williams & Wilkins, Philadelphia, PA.

Rowntree D (2000) *Statistics Without Tears: a primer for non-mathematicians* (2e). Penguin, Harmondsworth.

Saracci R (2010) *Epidemiology: a very short introduction*. Oxford University Press, Oxford.

Webb P and Bain C (2011) *Essential Epidemiology: an introduction for students and health professionals* (2e). Cambridge University Press, Cambridge.

Index

Entries in **bold** denote tables; entries in *italics* denote figures.